Live Longest Compendium

INTRODUCTION
WHAT WOULD YOU DO? WHO WOULD YOU CHOOSE?

If you went out to an airport and were offered two alternatives
1. A commercial aircraft which had flown for the last 30 years, at least, without an incident
2. An unregistered plane, built by someone with no qualifications, to their own design

As to the pilot
1. Someone with 30,000+ hours, combat experience, commercial training and license
2. Someone who is self-taught, without any qualifications or official training

Then, which plane and which pilot would you choose?

Even for the most stupid, most incompetent (see below) or most fervent believer in small enterprise, we all know the right answer. However, when it comes to health, more and more people, are opting for options 2.

A recent New York Times article pointed out how, in a paper published early this year (2019) in Nature Human Behavior, *those with the least understanding of science had the most science-opposed views, but thought they knew the most.* Lest anyone think this is only an American phenomenon, the study was also conducted in France and Germany, with similar results.

A small percentage of the public believes that vaccines are truly dangerous. People who hold this view — which is incorrect — also believe that they know more than experts about this topic. Many take vitamins and supplements, but the reasons are varied and are not linked to any hard evidence. Most of them say they are unaffected by claims from experts contradicting the claims of manufacturers. *Only a quarter said they would stop using supplements if experts said they were ineffective.* They must think they know better. I advise my patients, as well as in these books, as to the uselessness of manufactured vitamins and supplements and see their faint smile of disbelief and get the distinct impression many will continue to take them.

Part of this cognitive bias is related to the Dunning-Kruger effect, named for the two psychologists who wrote a seminal paper in 1999 entitled "Unskilled and Unaware of It." People who are the most incompetent (their word) believe they know much more than they do. A lack of knowledge leaves some without the contextual information necessary to recognize mistakes, they wrote, and their "incompetence robs them of the ability to realize it."

Bombarding people with more information about studies apparently isn't helping. How the information contained in them is disseminated and discussed may be much more important. This is why I have simplified my full books into this condensed Compendium. I'm afraid I was guilty of 'bombarding with studies.' Here now, however, I hope, are just the simplified essentials. If you want the studies, science and references then get the complete books.

And so it goes on: Rather than accessing the world's best medical and scientific trials by the world's proven best brains and universities, people are embracing instead the unqualified, zany, zealot world of *"wellness"* – their new religion. But as the commercial exploiters and scam artists compete this has now become dangerous as in *"extreme wellness"*.

This wellness industry is reputedly now worth $4.2 trillion world-wide with their 'recommendations' unusual and ever-more increasingly odd, with extremes of physical endurance, odd diets and supplement scams.

- The jade vagina eggs of Gwyneth Paltrow's Goop brand are now a notorious exposed scam
- Nootropics ('natural' or man-made supplements that are professed to boost memory and mental focus)
- Sweat lodges of hours in extremely hot enclosed spaces 'to purify group bodies and minds'
- Brrrn, the 'world's first cool-temperature fitness studio' in New York where people exercise in freezing conditions, so they lose more calories during a workout as the body shivers
- Flatline UK claims its workout are the hardest and most dangerous fitness class in the world with 45 minutes of high-intensity exercises, such as hoisting 60kg weights and sprinting for 45 metres – all in a 12kg weighted vest with just 15-second breaks. Paramedics are on hand during classes, and participants are required to sign a death waiver before getting started.
- Raw water, a derivative of the raw-food movement, recommends consuming water from springs or rivers without it being processed; devotees believe it is free of industrial toxins and rich in healthy microbes, which improve gut health. Health experts have stressed how most such water is contaminated from bird or animal dung with harmful bacteria, parasites and pesticides. But it's becoming more and more popular, with 2.5 gallons of untreated water costing $36.99 in the USA.
- Some if not all of these seize on an element of truth; saunas are beneficial, cold showers maybe, grass fed beef preferable and pure water mandatory, but they get it dreadfully wrong as they exploit their lemming followers with progressively bizarre and increasingly dangerous recommendations.

- And on and on and on, as these oh so willingly duped customers seek more and more extreme "wellness" fads to compensate for obvious personality problems and lack of knowledge.
- Also, of concern, are the extreme behaviours under the guise of sports, getting fit or conditioning. It has recently been found that fatalities among high school and college football athletes did not occur while playing the game of football, but rather during conditioning sessions, often associated with irrationally intense workouts, overexertion or punishment drills required by coaches and team staff.
- Perhaps we admire the ultra-marathon and marathon runners, but I have never known an elite athlete who has not had joint problems especially hip-replacements.

My favourite generation was those who fought in WW2. They witnessed the worst the world had to offer and had a bigger concept of life and great tolerance. Most people over 70 are stoic and are excellent patients when I operate on them. But thereafter it now falls off sequentially. Most Professionals I know from lawyers to other medical colleagues are exasperated by the 'Millennials' who seduced by TV plastic surgery or medical based programs expect unrealistic instant results and that modern medicine "should" supply them or a pill that cures everything.

Sadly, neither Governments nor the Medical Profession can provide this. Our genes only account for some 6% to 20% of our illnesses and premature deaths so **some 90% is up to you: You now have to look after yourself.**

IF you actually want the best medical evidence that has seen humans extend their lifespan from 27 years when Jesus preached to over 80 today, and if you want the *correct information* as to how to even improve on this…

then read on.

Caution: There is an emerging awareness that Lifespan is different to Healthspan. To that end I am reminded of the Greek myth of Eos and Tithonus to describe the difference. "The goddess Eos fell in love with a mortal man, Tithonus, and asked that he be granted eternal life, but forgot to ask for eternal youth. Tithonus lived forever but as a frail and immobile old man."

This whole Compendium / Series is to live longer-healthier combining both Life and Health Spans.

Dr Mileham Hayes

PREAMBLE

By the same logic as for selecting the best aircraft and pilot, who then is the best to ask for advice or help as to your health and living longer? Is it
- A 30-year-old, superb looking, fitness instructor?
- A celebrity selling their products?
- An Internet Vitamin and Supplement Site?
- A fat middle-aged Doctor?
- The Pharmacy or Health Shop with rows and rows of vitamins and supplements
- The Owner/Manager of a Spa, Health Ranch or Gym?
- Books by Authors who died before they achieved what their books claimed they would achieve
- A practicing medical Doctor who has spent a lifetime studying and researching the subject, is still consulting patients and operating, is healthy, fit and functioning, who, in other words, has "done it" and achieved it

OK: I am the latter (surprise! Surprise!). I still work in my clinic up to 12 hours a day. My Blood Pressure this morning is <130/70 and my pulse rate is <60 BPM. I take no medications. I bought some metformin but haven't taken any (see later). In other words I can claim to be living proof, so my research and advice must work, whereas most others are dubious in the extreme. I played sport and was physically active most of my life, but I can't say I am 'fit'. I am a Registered Specialist Physician / Internist ('Board Certified') and was appointed to the world's first Coronary Care Unit in 1968 which alerted me to the fact that Heart Attacks and Cardio-Vascular Disease was, and still is our greatest killers and I have monitored my Lipids and blood profiles for over 50 years.

For many years I was also a jazz musician (clarinet) and had my own radio and two national TV Programs and toured the world – not the healthiest lifestyle - but here I refer to the smoke in the jazz clubs, the late hours and not drugs which I abhor.

I am very happily married, we laugh a great deal, applaud the luck, success and good fortune of others. I have always had Labrador dogs, live in the country, love shopping and I garden – all things that are associated with living longer. But I have five kids which is associated with a shorter life (?!).

I am and have been very, very well aware of the things that are most likely to kill or disable us prematurely and have tried, while not being a saint or a zealot, to incorporate the evidence as the best medical research informs me which, over the years, has seen some contradicted but, all in all, it has been remarkably consistent and good. To that end I claim to be "living proof" as to the veracity of this, and now "my", advice.

By contrast, at my 50th Medical School Reunion I was the only one left from my group which included the Captain of Rugby, the Director of Psychiatry, an eminent Orthopaedic Surgeon, two GPs and my best friend. They were all either demented, dying or dead. (As one of the doctors I admire advised me "never go to reunions").

I gave up smoking in first year, have never eaten breakfast or lunch much and, trust me, I have lived life to the full. I once wrote an article, for the Nation's then leading magazine, on the "Best Restaurants in the World" as I investigated all the then, Three Star Michelin Guide French Restaurants, and I and my wife enjoy cooking but I have cut back on red meat and eat fish twice a week. I insidiously put on weight in the 90s but took it off (18kg) by researching how to do so (properly) and so wrote Slim 4 Life (Book 4 here).

I graduated from Queensland University which then had a very high and demanding standard, then to Sydney, Edinburgh and London where I specialised and was exposed to the best Medical Units and minds in the UK and, while offered some very flattering positions which may (or may not) have seen me 'rise' to being a pompous old fart, instead I returned to my less populated home town and lived on 12 acres on the outskirts. I now see it confirmed how the pollution in London (and all such densely populated cities) is killing people prematurely.

Luck, of course, plays a part. I should have been taken by sharks at least twice when, instead, one of my friends and the only other surfer, were. As a highly paid musician as well as a medical student I owned a Porsche 356a Speedster and practised 'low flying'. How I am not dead I would like to say was due to my skill, but it was luck, and this has made me acutely aware of our 'High Risk Behaviours' which we accept as normal lifestyles – but they are not.

I won't and can't say I have not been exposed to stress – try 120 hours a week running the Coronary Care Unit; my specialist exams when, of 300 Teaching Hospital Intellectual Elites, only 30 of us passed after three years of exams. Even now, the latest medical journals point out that clinicians suffer twice the burnout rate, then, when I told the Federated Liquor Trade Union thugs to perform an impossible and unnatural act, when they wanted me to 'unionise' our jazz club, such that they dobbed me into the Tax Office and every snide, dirty trick only they could resort to. But one learns from adversity and a little stress is good for us. However, in a new study (Biological Psychiatry May 09 2019) on newly graduated doctors, it was found that their telomeres (that prevent DNA cell damage) showed that their long hours, disrupted sleep and constant stress is damaging all the way down to their genes such that they age six times faster than normal. Remind me to write and thank my old hospitals and, for that matter, my old patients who called me at all hours to do house calls.

As to all that I am indebted to a Russian girlfriend and an old Trumpet playing friend and a Captain of Industry: I am a Scorpio and she explained to me that Scorpios have three parts to their nature: The Scorpion, The Elephant and the Eagle. The Scorpion part flicks his stinger over seeking immediate revenge; the Elephant never forgets and the Eagle the soars above and away. That sums me up perfectly, even if I don't believe in Astrology. And my friend advised me to use his Accountant to take care of the Taxation Office as 'he had been a POW on the Burma Railway and nothing frightens him'. He further advised me to 'let him worry about that and you get on practising medicine and playing your clarinet'. And he was right. We beat the bastards.

My Father was a very wise Doctor who predicted the deleterious effects of smoking in 1947 before anyone else. He also inculcated in me how he thought, in the 1920s, that it was "the refining of food that is the problem", that the char on steak was carcinogenic and to eat wholemeal bread. As he lived and practised through the discovery of vitamins, x-rays, antibiotics, organ transplants and most of the miracles modern medicine now offers, he had a perspective denied the modern doctor, such that hygiene, unpolluted air, a variety of fresh foods and keeping one's brain stimulated were important aspects to health that today's doctors and patients don't have time for. It's easier to take a pill.

I have seen the great years of medicine, but it is now altering with more and more interference, bureaucracy and (encouraged) litigation. Sadly, this is to the detriment of the patient.

I regarded medicine as 'The Nobel Profession' and as the most fascinating and rewarding (not financially) occupation. It is my passion. However, the practice of it has become increasingly unpleasant due to this political and bureaucratic interference such that, after a family history of some 300 years in medicine (one of my Grandfathers x times removed, was Physician the Prince Regent and granted Coat of Arms) I advised my bright son not to do it. He has no night calls, no tragedies, no worrying all night about the operation you just did and all he has to say is 'the mainframe went down'. As such, while medicine is now attracting the same best brains and dedicated people, it is also, by evolutionary necessity, developing a hardier race to resist these political-bureaucratic pathogens. More and more medical graduates will now, by necessity, retreat from clinical medicine having to see confrontational patients, and do research or hide away in a pathology lab or Radiology vault.

I do feel these books are a font of evidenced based, achievable, common sense to maximise our health and longevity at the current state of our knowledge. They represent my accumulated experience, if not my wisdom and, as I claim, I am 'living proof'. So far, so good, but I certainly don't know "what's around the corner".

References are to be found in the complete books should you want. Slim 4 Life was difficult to condense, and I would recommend the full book to those wanting to lose weight.

I do wish I had known and adopted all these recommendations 70 years ago and I would love to live another 50 years to see Diabetes 1 cured along with other auto-immune diseases and be astonished "So that was it!" when the causes are found.

LIVE LONGEST

COMPENDIUM

THE COMPLETE SERIES
in one abridged volume

The Five Absolute Basic Essentials to healthy longevity

1. **NEWTRITION**
   The Super-Mediterranean Diet

2. **SUCCESSFUL AGING**
   Stay fit, functioning and financial from childhood

3. **WHAT'S GOING TO KILL YOU THIS YEAR**
   The Missing Keys - avoiding the age specific killers

4. **SLIM 4 LIFE**
   Dieting alone is not enough: The 4 System medical program

5. **EXERCISE**
   Medically researched Exercise: Which and Why

by

Dr Mileham Hayes OAM, MB, BS (Qld), FRCP (Edin), FRCP (Lon).

Most health advice to live longer recommends diet, exercise, weight, no smoking and moderate drinking which is absolutely correct...but it needs fine tuning as there are some omissions.

**These 5 books do the fine tuning and fill in the omissions.
They are the culled essence of the world's best evidence presented in condensed, simplified versions.**

Emphasis has been placed on small, pleasant, achievable changes, substituting acceptable-to-you good habits, for any bad habits.

This Internet and Pop Age have opened the floodgates for odd, dubious and frankly dangerous mis-information. Scams abound.

How to Assess and Access the Best Health Information

Health information, but especially mis-information, is now ubiquitous, in books, magazines, talk shows, news stories, the media, but especially now, on the internet.

Does the information have

- A: *Authority*?
- B: Is there *Bias*?
- C: Is it *Complete and current*?

LIVE LONGEST

- A: *Authority*: Mileham Hayes is a Registered Specialist Physician with international experience. Only the world's best medical trials have been used.
- B: *Bias*: We all have bias but knowing this helps guard against it. Research that contradicts or challenges the author's bias is quoted as in the latest findings for pure fruit juice. Any bias and hypothesis against processed foods would seem increasingly supported by the latest research and findings.
- C: *Complete and current:* This Compendium is complete and current as at July 2019 accessing the 'Top 10' peer reviewed Medical Journals.

This Condensed Compendium of Live Longest five books provides you with the most complete information to maximize your health, prevent illnesses, live longest and healthiest. It presents just the essentials. It tells you what to do but doesn't go into the medical explanations (available in the full books along with references).

1. **NEWTRITION - The Super-Mediterranean Diet**
   - The world's most beneficial and healthiest foods
   - Recognized as the world's best diet – now updated
   - Incorporating Secrets of the Micronutrients

2. **SUCCESSFUL AGING - Staying Fit, Functional and Financial**
   - Starts in the womb but never too late
   - We are at our healthiest age 11 years
   - We stop growing around 18 years
   - We start to noticeably age at around 27 years
   - From 30 years we lose 1% of muscle each year
   - All illnesses start decades before we know it
   - Dementia is an epidemic
   - To prevent all these, START NOW!

3. **WHAT'S GOING TO KILL YOU THIS YEAR?**
   The Missing Keys - avoiding the age specific killers
   - There is something missing as with all the best health advice as to how live longest. This is "The Missing Keys"…the illnesses which predominantly occur at your present age
   - This book identifies these _and_ how to avoid them
   - Compression of Illnesses - 'Healthy Longer, sicker shorter'.
   - Who live longest and their lifestyles
   - Full Health Check recommendations

4. **SLIM 4 LIFE**
   - Not one diet suits everybody.
   - 4 different Programs are needed for successful weight loss
   - Diets
   - Nutrition
   - Behavior-Lifestyle changes
   - Exercise

5. **EXERCISE and PHYSICAL ACTIVITIES**
   - Which, why and how – the medical recommendations

TABLE OF CONTENTS

INTRODUCTION	iii
PREAMBLE	vii
A HEALTHY LONGER LIFE: The FIVE BASICS	1
BOOK 1 : NEWTRITION	9
The Micronutrient Plant (Phyto) Revolution	23
I Told You So	27
Unnatural: Processed, Refined Foods – Additives	37
Carbohydrates	49
BOOK 2 : SUCCESSFUL AGING	53
What Is Successful Aging	57
Age Changes: What To Expect (And Avoid)	61
Successful vs. Anti-Aging	73
Longevity & Life Expectancy	75
Staying Sharp	95
Dementia And Alzheimer Disease	101
Pollutants And Endocrine Disrupting Chemicals (EDC)	109
Medications	111
Sex	115
Preparing For Old Age: Begin In Your 40S.	119
Intimations Of Mortality: Momento Mori	123
BOOK 3 : WHAT'S GOING TO KILL YOU THIS YEAR?	125
SECTION A	129
What's Missing (To Allow Us Live Longer)?	131
Premature Deaths Overview	133
SECTION B	135
How To Use	137
Women	*139*
Overview	141

Young Women	143
Women Aged 25–44 Years	145
Women Aged 45–64 Years	149
Women 65 Years And Over	153
Men	*157*
Men Under 24 Years	159
Men 25–34 (44) Years	161
Men 35-44-64 Years	165
Men 65 Years And Over	171
SECTION C	175
The Missing Keys: Rationale	177
How To Best Use These Lists And Further Helpful Information	181
SECTION D	185
Who Lives The Longest	187
Life Begins At 40?	189
SECTION E	191
Premature Disabilities	193
Male And Female: Overall	195
What's Up, Doc?	197
SECTION F	201
Early Diagnosis & Treatment	203
Tests & Investigations	207
BOOK 4 : SLIM 4 LIFE	**217**
Why Are We So Fat?	225
How Do We Get Fat	227
Recommended Diets	229
Behaviour Modification	231
Motivation	233
Maintenance	237
The Benefits Of Weight Control	243
Slim 4 Life Key Essentials	245

BOOK 5 : EXERCISES & PHYSICAL ACTIVITIES   **247**

   Introduction   251
   The Best Medicine   255
   Definitions   257
   Exercise Types   261
   Planning   267
   Motivation   269
   HIIPA   273
   Exercise Programs   279
   Over 65s   295
   Some Age Changes = Exercise Deficiency   301
   Health Benefits   305
   Injuries   317
   Exercise And Weight   321

BOOK 1

NEWTRITION

The SUPER-MEDITERRANEAN

WORLD'S BEST DIET

NOTE:

Nutrition studies are, by necessity, observational. Randomized, controlled trials, the 'Gold Standard', to convincingly demonstrate benefits are unlikely, in fact impossible, to happen owing to the enormous cost of recruiting >100,000 participants and maintaining them on their respective diets for several years. However, meta-analyses at least provide a degree of evidence and certainty.

Newtrition has used only the best of these meta-analyses and studies.

The Medically Evidenced Most Beneficial Foods

ADVANCED CLEVER EATING

NEWTRITION *SUPER-MEDITERRANEAN* DIET BENEFITS

1. Lower All-Cause Mortality
2. 19 per cent reduced risk of early death
3. Less Heart Attacks and Strokes
4. Prevention of Cardiovascular Disease
5. Reduced Deaths in Patients with Cardiovascular Disease
6. Improved Post Heart Attack Survival
7. Low Inflammation, Coagulation, Triglycerides, raised HDL
8. Low Cholesterol & improved artery lining function
9. Reduced lipoprotein oxidation and LDL
10. Metabolic Syndrome halved
11. Slower Aging
12. Long Lasting Benefits
13. Less Total Cancer
14. Less Uterine Cancer
15. Less Breast Cancer Risk
16. Less Colorectal Cancer
17. Less Prostate cancer
18. Less Diabetes
19. Less Age Related Macular Degeneration (Blindness)
20. Brain Health and Protection – Slows Cognitive Decline
21. Less Alzheimer's
22. Less Depression
23. More Aged Physical Independence
24. Reduced Hip Fracture Risk in Women
25. Reduced Risk for Kidney Stones
26. Improved Survival of the Elderly
27. Less Chronic Obstructive Pulmonary Disease
28. Reduced Apnoea-Hypopnoea Index
29. Improved Erectile Dysfunction
30. Improved HDL
31. Further reduced risk Cancer, CVD, Premature Death
32. Improved Memory
33. Bigger Brain
34. Less Gout
35. Less Peripheral Artery Disease (PAD)
36. Higher muscle mass, bone density after menopause
37. Improves success of in vitro fertilization (IVF)
38. 25% sperm improvement
39. Improved Sleep
40. Improved Psoriasis
41. Increased Muscle Mass
42. Improved Endurance Exercise
43. Improved (less) Visceral damaging fat

Voted Best: Overall, Healthy Eating, Easiest to Follow, Best for Diabetes, Heart-Health and Best Plant-Based Diet in 2018 and 2019: U.S. News & World Report.

This SUPER-MEDITERRANEAN super-charges this even more.

A low-carb Mediterranean diet had a more significant effect on reducing visceral fat - fat around the liver, heart and pancreas, compared to low-fat diets with similar calorie counts. Moderate physical exercise reduced the degree of central abdominal obesity, a known risk factor for developing metabolic syndrome (associated with elevated blood pressure and cholesterol), and linked to increased risk of heart attack, stroke and peripheral artery disease (PAD).

In addition:
"Although sodium, sugar, and fat have been the main focus of diet policy debate in the past two decades, our assessment shows that the leading dietary risk factors for mortality are diets high in sodium, low in whole grains, low in fruit, low in nuts and seeds, low in vegetables, and low in omega-3 fatty acids."

SALT: An agreement to relax UK regulation of salt content in food is linked with *increasing cases of cardiovascular disease and gastric cancer*. In 2000 to 2001, mean salt intake was 10.5 g / day in men and 8.0 g / day in women and while this was falling due to mandatory restrictions this has been relaxed. Current guidelines are for 2.3g / day.

Both Governments and the Fast Food Industry either cannot, or will not, control your salt intake. It is up to you.

The NEWTRITION *SUPER-MEDITERRANEAN* DIET

Simply the best

20% Fruit
20% Vegetables
20% Grains, Seeds and Nuts
20% Protein - mostly plants
20% Superfoods (Micronutrients)

This is not some obsessional detailed daily measuring but rather a reminder to try and eat a variety of these five food groups every day (and avoid processed foods).

The Newtrition Superfoods:
Some foods have been identified as being richer in micronutrients and which donate greater benefits than others.

The Newtrition Superfoods are:
Apples/pears (white fruit), Apricots (dried), Beetroot, Berries, Celery, Cherries (esp. Montmorency), Chocolate-dark/cocoa, Citrus, Coffee, Fibre, Fish, Garlic/onion family, Grains (whole), Green Leafy Vegetables (esp. Bok Choy, Cabbage, Brocolli, Spinach), Inulin vegetables (chicory, leeks, asparagus, Jerusalem artichokes), Legumes, Nuts (walnuts, pecans, peanuts), Oats (barley) (rolled/cut), Olive Oil, Peppers Orange (Men), Prunes, Sweet Potato (purple), Vegetables green-yellow-cruciferous),

Maybe: Magnesium, Avocados, Curcumin, Cinnamon, Pomegranate Juice with Dates, Rosemary, Sage, Mankai duckweed, Mushrooms, Tomatoes, Vinegar, Apple Vinegar, Chamomile, Peppermint and Kombucha teas, Kefir (fermented milk)

Note: Pure fruit juice e.g. orange, have a high natural sugar content and, remarkably and disappointingly, have now been found to be associated with a higher rate of cancers. Eat the whole fruit as the fibre drags this sugar through and is good for you.

Chillies: While Chili consumption was found to be beneficial for body weight and blood pressure in previous studies, latest studies have noted faster cognitive decline in those who consistently ate more than 50 grams of chili a day. Memory decline was even more significant if the chili lovers were slim.

NEWTRITION DAILY ESSENTIALS

YES

1. Fruit variety, ensure berries, apples (skin), citrus
2. Veg: esp. green leafy, purple sweet potato, orange peppers (men), legumes and lentils
3. Nuts. 20g. walnuts, pecans, peanuts, almonds
4. Grains
5. Cocoa, Chocolate (dark)
6. Coffee
7. Extra Virgin Olive Oil (EVOO)
8. Fish
9. Fibre
10. Leave something on your plate: Never get full
11. Calm, pleasant meals. Happy people only
12. Superfoods

NO

1. Ultra-Processed foods or meats
2. Butter, cream
3. Added sugar
4. Sugar Sweetened Beverages (SSB) (sodas, soft drinks)
5. Pure fruit juice (whole fruit only)
6. Added salt
7. Vitamin supplements unless prescribed
8. Deep fried foods
9. No re-heated oil

WHAT NOT TO EAT

IS AS IMPORTANT AS

WHAT TO EAT

NEWTRITION'S WORLD'S BEST BREAKFAST

Breakfast is not necessary unless you feel you need it to function better, but it is not "the most important meal of the day".

1. Blueberries - for brain health
2. Granny Smith (skin) - gut health and stroke prevention
3. Walnuts, pecans - anti cancer, heart health.
4. Oats or Bran - lowers cholesterol, better microbiome
5. Grains - reduce All-Cause-Mortality, CVD and cancer
6. Flax (ground) - richest source Omega-3 ALA
7. Inulin - reduces visceral fat
8. Dried apricots. High potassium - lowers BP
9. Green bananas: Fiber speeds gut transit. Potassium
10. Biodynamic unsweetened yoghurt (< 4g sugar / 100g)
11. Fruit in season
12. Prunes - fibre / microbiome gut health
13. Coffee - Super-food

WORLD'S WORST BREAKFAST FOODS

1. Cereals high in sugar and salt
2. Sausages
3. Bacon/ham
4. Hash browns
5. Added salt
6. Butter
7. Crumpets, bagels, croissants
8. Waffles / Pancakes
9. Golden / Maple Syrup
10. Muffins
11. Sugar in your tea or coffee

NEWTRITION: Golden Rules

1. Do not worry about the occasional lapse or treat.
2. It is the long-term every-day ingestion that is harmful
3. Ensure great variety of freshest, local, ripest produce Benefits exceed any residual pesticides but wash
4. Pleasant, calm environment; enjoy your food & company
5. Eat slowly – it fills and satisfies you more
6. Don't eat until you feel full. Leave some food
7. No eating in cars. No Gas Station foods
8. "It's not what you cut out, it's what you replace it with". Do not replace fat with refined carbohydrates
9. Avoid all processed foods. Anything in a package is processed. All processing is bad until proven otherwise
10. Any label of ingredients you don't know means ultra-processed
11. No smoked, preserved (processed) meat (bacon, ham, sausages) and processed cheese.
12. Think more vegetarian
13. Vegetables every day esp. dark green leafy "cabbage" family
14. All fruit and vegetables are good, full of antioxidants Variety of fruit every day
15. Eat whole fruit, not just juice
16. The skin contains over 90% of the nutrients
17. Orange capsicums / peppers reduce Ca prostate
18. Berries x 3 times a week (slows cognitive decline)
19. An apple a day can reduce all-cause mortality, heart attacks and strokes. Oranges, pears too
20. Reduce potatoes (associated with hypertension)
21. Purple Sweet Potato / purple vegetables good
22. 15 g nuts daily. Less stroke & prostate cancer. Walnuts and pecans
23. Grains 70g/day lowers risk all-cause death, cancer, CVD
24. High-fiber reduces heart attacks, colorectal Ca (CAC)
25. Olive oil 20 ml / day. Reduced risk of stroke and CAD
26. Polyunsaturated oils the best for heart protection
27. No butter, no cream. Fermented dairy OK
28. Skim or "heart healthy" milk
29. Milk 200g, 50g cheese or 400 g dairy reduces risk of CAC
30. Every 300 mg Calcium (to 1900mg) reduces risk CAC
31. Eat more fish: X 2 a week. Avoid Fish Oil capsules.
32. Less red meat. All-cause mortality, Ca and CVD higher but best coronary arteries in the world were in meat eaters
33. No processed meat (bacon, ham, sausage)
34. Eat only organic poultry and eggs
35. More vinegar. Maybe a secret of the Mediterranean Diet
36. More fresh herbs, garlic
37. Chilies lower risk of total mortality and Ca risk

38. Breakfast cereals of oats best. Avoid commercial processed brands. Breakfast is not necessary
39. A glass of red wine with food daily. Women with family history of breast Ca or men who smoke should abstain
40. Coffee 4 cups a day. Green or no-milk tea
41. Dark chocolate or 2 heap teaspoons cocoa, daily
42. Reduce Salt: Current guidelines are for 2.3g / day. Check labels
43. Taste before you add salt; break the "autopilot" habit
44. Increase potassium: fruits (dried apricots)
45. Reduce sugar intake < 4 g sugar per 100 g in any serving
46. Avoid HFCS (High Fructose Corn Syrup in many drinks)
47. Micro-filtered water (to avoid Giardia & Cryptosporidium).
48. Don't shop hungry. No portion distortion, small, no 2nds
49. Dry bake vegetables or microwave.
50. Avoid soya bean oil may increase obesity and diabetes.
51. Microwaving veg best preserves vitamins and minerals
52. Avoid the middle aisles in supermarkets.
53. No very hot beverages (carcinogenic to throat)
54. Intermittent Fasting Diets for health and weight loss
55. Pomegranate juice + 3 dates

Bar the Char

Charred, smoked, and well-done meat could raise cancer risk—pancreatic, colorectal, and prostate cancers, in particular. Heterocyclic amines (HCAs) or heterocyclic aromatic amines (HAAs), are a class of chemical that forms in cooked red meat and, to a lesser extent, in poultry and fish. high intake of well-done meat and high exposure to meat carcinogens, particularly HCAs, may increase the risk of human cancer

No More Squeezed Orange Juice

An increase in sugary drink consumption, including 100% fruit juices and other sugary drinks, both were positively associated with the risk of overall cancer and breast cancer. In contrast, no association was detected between artificially sweetened beverage consumption.
This is disappointing to those of us who thought a glass of 'freshly squeezed orange juice' was healthy. Although elsewhere I point out how the whole orange should be eaten to get the fibre and to drag through the sugar,

Yoghurt

Men who eat at least two servings a week of yogurt may be lowering their risk for colorectal cancer. Compared to men who didn't eat any yogurt, those who had at least two servings weekly were 19% less likely to develop conventional adenomas and 26% less likely to develop adenomas with the highest malignant potential.

CHAPTER 1.

THE MICRONUTRIENT PLANT (PHYTO) REVOLUTION

The discovery of the **_MACRO_-nutrients** of *1. protein, 2. carbohydrates and 3. fats and oils,* has led to exhaustive studies as to their functions, benefits and possible deleterious effects, such as elevating cholesterol, and to on-going debates as to the best ratios and the best fats (oils).

The importance of the **_MICRO_-nutrients** became evident with the discovery of *vitamins, minerals and amino acids* many of which are essential. But even then, we do not know the full spectrum of what some, such as magnesium, contribute.

But, as well as these vitamin and mineral micronutrients about which, in the main, we know a great deal, there are also thousands of **Phytochemicals** in our foods about which we know very little.
Phyto is Greek for "plant" and these thousands of micro-chemicals are mostly plant based. There are a few micronutrients that are animal based - but only a few. And while the lack of a vitamin or a mineral may result in a devastating disease, which makes its function obvious and essential to life, the phytochemicals and other micronutrients are not essential to life and are an evolving mystery.

A mystery, however, that is just being unlocked.

There are good foods that donate health benefits and there are bad foods that damage and shorten our lives.

For some reason certain foods seem to be beneficial while others can cause rashes, severe allergies, make us ill, send us on mind-bending "trips" or even poison us. But some seem to reduce and maybe prevent, not only our two greatest killers, Cardiovascular Disease and Cancer but many other illnesses as well.
As a whole family they are grouped as "Phytochemicals" but the beneficial ones are classified as **phyto-_nutrients._**

Protein, carbs and fat are essential, but these other preventive benefits do not seem to be derived from them, nor from the vitamins, minerals or the amino acids, which contribute to our health in more dramatic "essential" ways (no vitamin B12 etc - we die).

However, while not "essential", these micro (phyto) nutrient's benefits are profound and include: Improved All-Cause Mortality, Less Heart Attacks and Strokes, Prevention of Cardiovascular Disease, Halving the Metabolic Syndrome, Slower Aging, Less Total Cancer, Less Diabetes, Less Dementia/Alzheimer's, Less Depression, Improvement of erectile dysfunction, Further, Reduction of Premature Death.

Caution: However, when synthetic vitamins and minerals or phytonutrients are then added (replaced) to processed or junk foods they don't provide the same benefits, nor do they when taken as a pill or supplement (unless you have a diagnosed deficiency or need).

Fresh plants are necessary, and also, as no one ingredient or plant can provide all the benefits and as no one such special plant or ingredient can be found, then it must be the amalgamation, the variety, the diversity, the array, the complete spectrum and combination of all the ingredients from different foods working in a symbiotic partnership.

It must therefore be necessary to consume a *variety of plants (fruit and vegetables)*.

All the best diets were based on the Traditional Mediterranean Diet. And recent research of some 2,000,000 people, has found yet even more benefits if we eat more of certain food groups which provide these phytonutrients.

But the benefits from eating as well as possible via the Newtrition Super-Mediterranean Diet will nevertheless be nullified if processed food is also eaten. My analogy to this is that "By breathing fresh mountain air you cannot continue to smoke...by eating the beneficial foods you cannot continue to eat processed foods".

There are also some single foods or family of foods do seem to have "super" qualities: "Green leafy vegetables" seem to be good for our gut and reduce cancer of the colon. Coffee has been called the "ultimate super-food" reducing all-cause-mortality, cardiovascular disease, diabetes, cancers, depression and maybe Alzheimer's and many more. Coffee contains more than 1,000 chemical compounds yet, despite it being the most consumed beverage in the world, less than 30 of these 1,000 compounds have been subjected to juried, health related research.

As far as is now known I have listed these in the Newtrition Foods.

As it took centuries for the vitamins to be recognised and their every-day ingestion to be recognized as essential, this is where we are at today with the phytochemicals. Eventually, but a long way away, no doubt a specific phyto will be found to provide specific benefits such as prevention of atheroma-heart attacks or prevention of cancer of the colon or even Alzheimer's

Disease but until then *it doesn't really matter because all we have to do is eat them now - we don't have to know how they work!*

The orange has more vitamin C than any other citrus, but it also has some 69 other ingredients or phytochemicals. We humans have been evolving on this planet for some 2.7 million years. We can't make vitamin C, so we had to find foods that did. Now, you don't have to be Einstein, who didn't know much or anything about vitamin C or Linus Pauling who invented the Pill and thought he did, to wonder, as I have, "what are these other 69 nutrients doing?" They are not just there to give colour or flavour, although some do. What then? Surely, it is just plain common sense that they help our gut better absorb the Vitamin C and then speed it more efficiently throughout our bodies' metabolic chains? And, in fact, this has already been shown to be the case.

So what are the other 5,000 flavenoids and the thousands of other nutrients doing? We need them from different foods to mix with each other to provide this amazing protection and enhancement to our health.

There are only 13 vitamins and the drug companies push "multivitamin" supplements unmercifully with no evidence as to benefit. There are only 13 vitamins but there are over 5000 phytochemicals.

Welcome to the Micronutrient Revolution.

CHAPTER 2.
I TOLD YOU SO

Since the first (sold out) edition of my book "Newtrition" it is gratifying, but not surprising, to find my recommendations now confirmed in eight large subsequent surveys.

First, one of the largest surveys of data on global dietary habits and longevity which covered 195 different countries from 1990 to 2017. This survey found that consuming vegetables, fruit, fish and whole grains was strongly associated with a longer life — and that people who skimped on such healthy foods were more likely to die before their time. The study, published in The Lancet, 3rd April 2019, concluded that one-fifth of deaths around the world were associated with poor diets — defined as those short on fresh vegetables, seeds and nuts but heavy in sugar, salt and trans fats.

Second, it was estimated that 11 million deaths that could have been avoided. Most of those, around 10 million, were from cardiovascular disease. The next biggest diet-related killers were cancer, with 913,000 deaths, and Type 2 diabetes, which claimed 339,000 lives.
I would again make the claim that, given these and the other studies (as detailed in the full book), the Newtrition Super-Mediterranean Diet is the healthiest.

Third, further, as now emphasised in Book 4, **Slim 4 Life** and later here, the eating of processed foods is also very detrimental as, again gratifyingly, this has also been confirmed by a French study, published late 2018, of some 45,000 people which found for the first time a link between the consumption of ultra-processed foods, characterized as ready-to-eat or ready-to-heat formulations and a higher risk of death with just a 10 percent increase in the proportion of ultra-processed foods in the diet corresponded to a 15 percent increase in mortality.
Basic advice is to avoid food and drinks listing multiple complex chemicals on their labels.

Fourth, in 2018, the same study, observed more cancers among heavy consumers of these foods. The question remains, what is it about these foods that causes negative impacts on health? One popular hypothesis is the presence of additives.

Fifth, my emphasis on fibre has also been supported. "The evidence from prospective studies is remarkably consistent that a higher intake of fiber is related to lower risk of type 2 diabetes, cardiovascular disease and weight gain," Dr. Walter Willett, professor of nutrition and epidemiology at Harvard School of Public Health 2019.

Sixth, a decade long study of more than 30,000 people, published in April, 2019, in the most respected Annals of Internal Medicine, found that certain vitamins and minerals may help extend your life and keep you from dying of cardiovascular disease – *but only if you get those beneficial nutrients from foods, not supplements or pills.*

Seventh, Autism: molecular changes that happen when neural stem cells are exposed to high levels of an acid commonly found in processed foods have been identified. In a study published June 19, 2019, in *Scientific Reports*, scientists discovered how high levels of Propionic Acid (PPA), used to increase the shelf life of packaged foods and inhibit mold in commercially processed cheese and bread, reduce the development of neurons in fetal brains. The combination of reduced neurons and damaged pathways impede the brain's ability to communicate, resulting in behaviours that are often found in children with autism.

Eighth, the "umbrella review," appearing in the *Annals of Internal Medicine*, the best data surrounding vitamins and supplements in one place, in a comprehensive report of randomized trials that examined their effects on cardiovascular disease and overall mortality.

After analysing nearly 300 trials and one million participants, the conclusions are that ***there is no high-quality evidence that any vitamin pill or supplement has a beneficial effect on overall mortality.***

Vitamin or Supplement	Patients number tested	Benefit(s): Harm
Anti-oxidants	992,129	Nothing, zilch, blot
Beta carotene		Nil
Calcium		Nil
Calcium +Vitamin D		Increased stroke risk
Folic acid		Nil
Iron		Nil
Multivitamins		Nil
Omega-3 fatty acids		Nil
Selenium		Nil
Vitamin A		Nil
Vitamin B complex		Nil
Vitamin B6		Nil
Vitamin B3 - niacin		Nil
Vitamin C		Nil
Vitamin D		Nil

And while this analysis didn't record vitamin E other studies have shown Vitamin E is potentially unsafe if taken by mouth in high doses. If you have a condition such as heart disease or diabetes, do not take doses of 400 IU/day or more. Some research suggests that high doses might increase the chance of death and possibly cause other serious side effects.

Vitamins and supplements are only for (proven) deficiency states, such as third-world countries or old people eating poorly. 'Normal' people on normal diets derive NO benefits. But hey! Don't believe the world's best non-profit, independent medical and scientific studies and evidence! Keep reading and believing the Internet Blogs of the unqualified or the Looney Zealots. Made in China at incredible mark-ups...just for you.

I am not being supercilious here. It is very, _very_ hard, for any of us, not to be conned and convinced by the vitamin and supplement industry. They have massive amounts of money ($Billions if not $Trillions) to convince us that we need their products and that 'just food' isn't enough. But, what is worse, they then prey on vulnerable people's fears, such as old people worried about dementia and they push their useless 'brain boosting' supplements. So what I am trying to do is to reassure you that you don't need any and to highlight the fact that these vitamins and supplements are made in dubious, unknown factories, usually in China, are frequently found not to contain what they claim or even contain banned or damaging ingredients...and, the madness is they claim these synthetic, dubious factory ingredients are better than the natural food humans have evolved to metabolise. Artificial or synthetic vitamins and supplements don't work in human bodies but are just urinated out.

I know this wont convince the body-builders, the gym-junkies, the elite athletes but, while I won't say they have major mental problems they do often have an image problem (the "walnuts in a condom" body-builders look) or they desperately seek an edge over their competition and so are ripe for any nutritional, let alone supplement boost.

As most if not all are just voided they do no harm but most are unregulated and untested and steroids, heavy metals and other toxins have been found in them or, as with fish oil capsules, didn't contain the amounts they claimed (that's OK fish oil doesn't help the heart anyhow).

If people taking vitamins and supplements feel better, it is because they
    a.   Are leading a healthier life anyway
    b.   The Placebo Effect
    c.   Retail Therapy Syndrome: Spend, swallow and feel better

They have best been described as "pseudoscientific 'wellness' profiteering." They are a waste of your money and an insult to anyone's intelligence but a remarkable marketing exercise. Don't be duped.

The Newtrition Super-Mediterranean Foods give you all the vitamins and supplements you need in the correct dose, better absorbed and better metabolized or utilized by our bodies. The money you now waste on these can buy better, fresher and more varied foods.

Predictions Come True
Do I feel smug at predicting all these? Not really, as the evidence has been there for anyone to access (but the Vitamin and Fast Food Industries make it difficult and saturate advertising the market). But it's nice to have more and more excellent trails and studies confirming my 'predictions'. Rather, I feel frustrated that every day I still examine patients who are taking vitamins and supplements "just in case" when all they are doing is overloading their now very expensive urine and funding a $30 billion rip-off scam called the Vitamin Industry. And, when I check out the Supermarkets, I am horrified at the trolleys full of soft drink/sodas, chocolates and sweets, packaged foods, biscuits, cookies, cakes, heat and eat meals, processed junk and yes vitamins, but singularly sparse, if any, as to fruit and vegetables – the actual best source of vitamins and micronutrients. Most of the people with these junk trolleys are fat or distinctly unhealthy looking. I am not being cynical to point out they are pushing their own premature illness and death trolleys.

In addition
Low Sperm Counts: A Western junk food diet — high in processed and red meats, refined grains, chips, and sweets — is associated with lower sperm count and overall impaired testicular function, according to a talk given at the annual conference of the European Society for Human Reproduction and Embryology held in Vienna June 2019.

Diet and Cancer Prevention
Diet has an important role to play in cancer prevention. While there are no miracle foods, an overall healthy diet is an important cancer-prevention goal.

According to the World Cancer Research Fund (WCRF), 20 percent of all cancers diagnosed in the U.S. are related to poor dietary choices and lack of exercise.

Cancer cases were associated with overconsumption of certain foods and sweetened beverages, as well as low intake of important nutrients and minerals, namely low whole grain intake, low dairy intake, high processed meats intake, low vegetable intake, low fruit intake, high red meat intake, high intake of sugar-sweetened beverages.

The Continuous Update Project (CUP), an ongoing review of research on nutrition and cancer conducted by the WCRF and the American Institute for Cancer Research (AICR), is helping to clarify the diet-cancer interaction. To date, the CUP has found evidence that diet, weight, and physical activity level can impact risk of 17 cancers, including colorectal, breast, mouth, pharynx, larynx, oesophageal, stomach, bladder, kidney, liver, gallbladder, ovarian, prostate, endometrial, pancreatic, and lung cancers. Being overweight or obese is clearly linked with an increased risk of 13 of these cancers and seven in 10 Americans are now overweight or obese as is the case in most Western countries.

Increased Cancer Risk:
CAC Cancer of the Colon) / CRC (Colon Rectal Cancer)
Medscape July 11, 2019
"Red meat, processed meat, and alcohol".

Improved Risk
Physical activity was associated with a reduction in the risk for incident colon cancer of slightly more than 20% but not protective against rectal cancer.

Fiber from bread and cereals lowered the risk.

Worse Risk
The World Health Organization classifies processed meat as carcinogenic and red meat as probably carcinogenic,.
People who eat red and processed meat 4 or more times a week have a higher risk of developing bowel cancer than those who eat red and processed meat less than twice a week.

Preserved Meat
Increasing processed meat consumption by the equivalent of 1 strip of bacon or 1 slice of ham per day was associated with a 19% higher risk for CRC.

Red Meat
Similarly, increasing daily red meat intake by the equivalent of 1 thick slice of roast beef was associated with an 18% increase in the risk for CRC.

Alcohol
Alcohol consumption also raised the risk for CRC. drinking 2 or more alcoholic beverages per day. On the flip side, eating whole grains daily and ramping up activity levels can reduce the risk.

Hazard Ratio (HR) for each 10-g/day increment of alcohol from Beer was 1.11. Wine was 1.05; Spirits was 1.08.

A hazard ratio of 3 means that three times the number of events are seen in the treatment group at any point in time. A hazard ratio of 0.333 tells you that the hazard rate in the treatment group is one third of that in the control group.

No Effect
Intakes of poultry, cheese, tea, and coffee. fruit and vegetable fiber were not associated with risk for CRC.

I have long advocated eating green leafy vegetables to prevent CRC so this is disappointing but, "just in case", here is the following, why not?

- Diets high in fruit *may* lower risk of stomach and lung cancer.
- Eating vegetables containing carotenoids, such as carrots, Brussels sprouts, and squash, *may* reduce the risk of lung, mouth, pharynx, and larynx cancers.
- Diets high in non-starchy vegetables, like broccoli, spinach, and beans, *may* help protect against stomach / oesophageal cancer.
- Eating oranges, berries, peas, bell peppers, dark leafy greens high in vitamin C *may* also protect against oesophageal cancer.
- Foods high in lycopene, such as tomatoes, guava, and watermelon, *may* lower the risk of prostate cancer.

Processed meats (such as ham, deli meats, bacon, salami, hot dogs, and sausages) often have added nitrates, which are associated with increased colorectal and stomach cancer risk. Meats labeled "no nitrates added" are often made with "natural" sources of nitrate, such as celery juice, and so also are not nitrate free. Eating smoked or salt-cured meats also increases exposure to potential cancer-causing agents. Intake of processed meats should be eliminated or reduced.

Americans have not appreciably changed their consumption of processed meats during the last 18 years, despite growing evidence linking luncheon meats, sausage, hot dogs, bacon, and other processed meats to illnesses such as colorectal cancer, an analysis of survey data has found. Fish and shellfish consumption also did not change: fewer than 15% of US adults met the recommended intake of 8 ounces per week.

During the same period, poultry consumption increased whereas consumption of unprocessed red meat — including beef, pork, and lamb — did show a downward trend. One fourth of American adults still eat more than the recommended weekly limit for red meat of 500 grams, or fewer than three servings, however.

Red meat (meat from any mammal, including beef, veal, pork, lamb, mutton, horse, and goat) has been associated with increased risk of colon cancer. But the latest study (above) found poultry was OK.
Cooking meat at very high temperatures (such as frying, broiling, or grilling) can lead to the formation of chemicals that might increase cancer risk. Try braising, steaming, poaching, stewing, and microwaving meats instead.

Alcoholic beverages are associated with increased risk of mouth, pharynx, larynx, esophageal, breast, colorectal, stomach, and liver cancers. Cutting out or reducing alcohol intake could lower the number of cancer cases, especially for breast cancer.

Pesticides, herbicides, genetic modification, and irradiation on foods have not been proven to either increase or decrease cancer risk. Overwhelming scientific evidence supports the overall health benefits and cancer-protective effects of eating vegetables and fruits, so the benefits of eating these foods far outweigh any potential risk. Wash fresh fruits and vegetables thoroughly before eating (even organics), to lower exposure to chemicals and to limit the risk of health effects from germs. No data to date support concerns about cancer and genetically modified organisms (GMOs).

Decreasing Cancer Risk:
There are no magic foods that, when added to one's diet, will prevent cancer, but there is good evidence that an overall healthy dietary pattern rich in plant foods can help to lower risk. Plant foods (fruits, vegetables, whole grains, legumes, nuts, and seeds) are rich in fibre, vitamins, minerals, and phytochemicals, all of which have roles to play in health. Some of these plant compounds act as antioxidants, which reduce potentially-carcinogenic damage to cells caused by normal chemical reactions in the body.

Whole grains. Research shows an association between diets high in *whole grains* (and low in refined-processed grains) and lower risk of colorectal cancer. Refined-grain foods are no good such as most breakfast 'cereals.' They are high-sugar and linked to weight gain,

Fruits and vegetables. According to the American Cancer Society (ACS), scientific evidence suggests that eating vegetables and fruits is associated with lower risk of several types of cancer, including cancers of the lung, mouth, throat, larynx, oesophagus, stomach, colon, and rectum. Again this is 'suggestive' and lacks definite evidence.

There is no proof at this time that a strict vegetarian or vegan diet is any better at reducing cancer risk than simply reducing intake of red and processed meats. Additionally, not all plant-based diets are equal. Studies suggest that the quality of the plant foods we consume matters more than simply eliminating animal foods from the diet. High intake of fruits, vegetables, and whole grains is associated with health benefits, whereas high intake of unhealthy 'plant-based foods' that are low in fiber or high in added sugars is not. A plant-based dietary pattern appears to be beneficial for preventing not only cancer but also diabetes and heart disease.

Skip the Supplements: Eating nutrient-rich foods (like vegetables, fruits, and other plant-based foods) may reduce cancer risk but taking dietary supplements does not have the same effect. Antioxidants, for example, may have anti-cancer activity, but consuming antioxidants in the form of dietary supplements is not associated with reduced cancer risk. In some cases, there is evidence of possible harm from getting nutrients from supplements as opposed to from foods. High doses of the vitamin A precursor beta-carotene, vitamin E, and folate have each been linked with an increased risk of certain cancers. According to preliminary research reported by the ACS, Vitamin D may help prevent colorectal cancer, but results from large studies won't be ready for several years. Don't rely on supplements for cancer prevention.

Protein Shakes – Beware
Protein supplements have long been the trend among health and fitness conscious millennials but protein shakes can be very calorie heavy and can also contain additives which may have side-effects and could be doing as much damage to your waistline as a Big Mac and by adding two scoops of protein to your milk. Best to get from lean meat and fish.

Brain Boosting Supplements- another scam
These prey on people who fear Alzheimer's but Evidence-based review examined current efficacy data of brain-health supplements and concluded that they could not endorse any ingredient, product, or supplement formulation designed for brain health, but they did endorse a healthy diet as an alternative.

Beware the "Psychedelic Renaissance"
I inform you of this only to condemn it in the strongest way.
The practice of micro-dosing — taking about a tenth of a party dose of LSD and other mind-altering drugs as a kind of mental tonic — is, apparently, all the rage in the tech community. The niche trend is now a mainstream craze and American GQ magazine declared that what started as a "body-tinkering, mind-hacking, supplement-taking productivity craze in Silicon Valley is now spreading to more respectable workplaces" - all in the name of self-improvement.

Firstly, Einstein, Newton, Faraday, Shakespeare, Leonardo and all such assembled geniuses did not need any such 'boost' – so, if you ain't got it no drug is going to improve your IQ or creativity. Secondly, the long-term effects are simply unknown, and your family may not like having to care for as paranoid, gibbering idiot.

Why humans love taking drugs must be deep in our DNA...maybe it's because we can. But, before a legitimate drug can be prescribed it has to go through many, many trials and tests and then be purified into known ingredients and dose. Whereas these are not regulated or tested, and no analytical dose guaranteed. A 'recipe' for disaster.

VITAMIN PILLS AND SUPPLEMENTS ARE A SCAM

(Unless you have a *proven* deficiency or a very poor diet)

Do not trust the "Health" shop. Do not listen to any advice other than a qualified medical practitioner and even then, I'd be cautious if he, or she, was "alternate"

EAT THE NEWTRITION SUPER-MEDITERRANEAN FOODS

They provide ALL nutritional needs AND donate health benefits

There are only 13 vitamins but today there are over 87,000 "supplements" on the market. Most have not been tested and most have dubious, if any, benefit. Whereas a variety of fresh food provides all, in the right dose and more efficiently absorbed and metabolised.

WE CANNOT PROCESS PROCESSED FOODS

CHAPTER 3.

UNNATURAL: PROCESSED, REFINED FOODS – ADDITIVES

Ultra-processed food is a concept devised by the Brazilian nutrition researcher Carlos Monteiro. As of 2018 the concept is loose and evolving.

Monteiro uses the term to refer to the processing of substances derived from foods baking, frying, extruding, molding, hydrogenation and hydrolysis and several transformation processes including heating at high temperatures and the presence of additives, emulsifiers and texturizers. Many ready-to-heat products that are rich in salt or sugar and low in vitamins and fibre fall under this category.

They generally include a large number of additives such as preservatives, sweeteners, sensory enhancers, colorants, flavors and processing aids, but little or no whole food. They may be fortified with micronutrients. The aim is to create durable, convenient and palatable ready-to-eat or ready-to-heat food products suitable to be consumed as snacks or to replace freshly prepared food-based dishes and meals.

There would seem to be a distinction between 'ultra-processed' and 'processed' when the latter refers to minimal interference such as tinned tomatoes or using just salt as a preservative as with proscuito.

As classified by the NOVA Food Classification System developed at the University of Sao Paulo in Brazil, "ultra-processed food and beverages" "are industrial formulations made entirely or mostly from substances extracted from foods (oils, fats, sugar, starch and proteins). They are derived from hydrogenated fats and modified starch and synthesized in laboratories.

Scientists analyzed 230,156 products and found 71% of products such as bread, salad dressings, snack foods, sweets, sugary drinks and more were ultra-processed. Among the top 25 manufacturers by sales volume, 86% of products were classified as ultra-processed. Bread and bakery products were consistently among the highest.

Refining of Grains

The refining of grains wherein the husk is removed stripping out all the vitamins and micro-nutrients and referred to as 'refining' is, to me, ultra-processing.

> AUTHOR'S NOTE: The terms Refined, Processed and Ultra-Processed are essentially the same. Additives, preservatives, colorants, enriched or any chemicals whatsoever should be regarded with suspicion.

Refining consists of when the bran and germ are stripped off all that is left is nutrient poor starch in the form of white (Processed) flour. Grains were originally refined to extend its shelf life. However, Grains consist of fibre-rich bran and nutrient-vitamin rich germ, which is lost in the refining.

Wheat is the most eaten grain in Western diets and 98% of this wheat is eaten in the form of processed white flour.

% of Nutrients Lost by Refining

	loss
Protein	25%
Fibre	95%
Calcium	56%
Copper	62%
Iron	84%
Manganese	82%
Phosphorous	69%
Potassium	74%
Selenium	52%
Zinc	76%
Vitamin B1	73%
Vitamin B2	81%
Vitamin B3	80%
Vitamin B5	56%
Vitamin B6	87%
Folate	59%
Vitamin E	95%

'Enriching' only chemically adds 5 of the lost 25 nutrients back!?

I contend that it is these ultra-processed foods that have caused the current epidemic of obesity as obesity shadowed their introduction after WW2. It is fashionable to blame our genes or now our gut microbiome *but these have not changed – only our food has.*

And so they have for all of us with obesity now an official epidemic causing its downstream effects of the 'Diseases of Affluence' of Hypertension, Heart Attacks, Strokes, Diabetes 2, Arthritis, Depression and so many more. I also wonder about the new increase in Colorectal Cancers in younger people (<50 yrs) which defies all trends.

Sometimes we can't see the wood for the trees and although I suspect some of my colleagues are reaching the same conclusions, no one else has come out and accused Ultra-processed and Refined Foods as the cause of our obesity epidemic.

Of course, we have to over-eat too but the affordability of junk food (three times cheaper than fruit and veg), it's convenience (24 hrs a day, 7 days a week and home delivered) or its delicious taste designed to hit our 'bliss spot', make over-eating junk food so much easier and hence we are overeating. Americans eat an extra 788 calories a day when only 20 more will make us fat, but I also suspect, these additives are so new and untested, we simply can metabolise them as we do foods we have evolved 2 to 5 million years to eat and these cause an unrecognised 'cascade' corrupting our normal, evolved metabolic pathways, jam them up and divert them to lay down fat.

Our food, this ultra-processed food has evolved faster in the last 60 years than the previous 60,000 (or even 600,000) years.
Go figure.

Processed Cascade
The problem with foods that make people fat isn't all caused in that they have too many calories, but also, it's that they cause a cascade of reactions in the body that promote fat storage and make people overeat. Processed carbohydrates—foods like chips, sugar-soda/soft drinks, crackers/cakes/biscuits, and even white rice—digest quickly into sugar and increase levels of the hormone insulin.

Avoid Food Bloggers
Out of nine leading UK weight management blogs only one was trustworthy. It was the only one by an accredited nutritionist whereas most bloggers had no relevant qualifications, their blogs lacked credibility and included unhealthy recipes. European Conference Obesity 2019.

WARNINGS and EXPLANATIONS

All food trials and studies are essentially *observational*. Certainly, we can remove vitamin C and induce scurvy and then cure it by re-introducing vitamin C but we can't do it with say bananas, fish or meat.
What can be done, however, is to *observe* the diets of those people live longer. In essence these are people who eat a variety of fresh foods, don't eat factory – processed foods and who are also physically active.

Food studies are ripe (pun intended) with confounders. A confounder is something, other than the thing being studied, that could be causing the results seen in a study.

Hence the vegetarians and vegans can claim their diet is the healthiest as they are leaner and live longer. But to then extrapolate that meat is bad is spurious (the healthiest coronary arteries so far are in meat eaters and the human race would have self-exterminated had they been vegetarians). But further, vegetarians and vegans are 'food obsessed' as part of their overall health obsession and invariably lead a healthier lifestyle of no smoking, no booze and keeping trim. If you add some grass-fed meat to this, as in twin studies, there is no real difference.

Vegans and vegetarians are leaner and live longer because they have a strict code across the whole spectrum of lifestyles. Most do not smoke, do not drink alcohol, let alone sugary pop, and the religious ones, such as the Adventists, support each other socially. All of which promote longevity.

The opposite confounders are the Good Ol' Boys who char their steaks while smoking, drinking, eating sausages and junk food and who are invariably overweight and sedentary, all of which reduce lifespans. Hence it can again be spuriously claimed that all meat is bad.

There would also seem to be a sinister side to vegetarian promotions in that they own much of the breakfast cereal market, the nut farms of California and they have infiltrated and funded many of the Dietician Associations. But that's OK, Coke helps fund the American Cardiology Association.

There is also the trap that we all fall into - personal bias. Cholesterol was "bad". And so it is – the Low Density (small molecule) LDL - which are just plaque forming waste products. Same with fats. Now there are good and bad.

In addition: John Ionaddis, MD, has been particularly vocal about these limitations, writing: "*A large majority of human nutrition research uses nonrandomized observational designs, but this has led to little reliable progress. This is mostly due to many* epistemologic *problems, the most*

important of which are as follows: difficulty detecting small (or even tiny) effect sizes reliably for nutritional risk factors and nutrition-related interventions; difficulty properly accounting for massive confounding among many nutrients, clinical outcomes, and other variables; difficulty measuring diet accurately; and suboptimal research reporting. Tiny effect sizes and massive confounding are largely unfixable *problems that narrowly confine the scenarios in which nonrandomized observational research is useful."*
I agree with this.

NEWTRITION has no vested interests or trying to convert you to a cult. Neither has God spoken to me personally to advise me as to what to eat. Instead the world's best independent trials have been consulted and, while the above observational limitations are acknowledged, it is equally obvious that we are the fattest humans in history, there is an increasing epidemic of obesity and heart disease and cancer are our two biggest killers. And good nutrition and not eating bad foods (processed, preserved, additives deep fried in old oil and so on) would seem to reduce both of these killers.

This Diet is unashamedly based on the Mediterranean Diet, now recognised by the WHO as 'the best' but I have now distilled, augmented and updated it as NEWTRITION the Super-Mediterranean Diet.

In 1997, much to the delight of the Fast Food Industry, they found that *'consumers (had) dropped all pretence of wanting healthy food'*

Poor diet (world-wide) is consistently responsible for more disease and death than physical inactivity, smoking and alcohol combined.

Americans now spend more on fast food than on higher education, personal computers, software or new cars and more on fast food than on movies, books, magazines, newspapers, videos and recorded music – combined.

Around 15,000 years ago humans ate around 150 ingredients a week. Today we mostly only eat 20, most of which are processed – refined.

Our food has changed more in the last 60 years than the previous 60,000o years. Since World War 2 there have been more than 80,000 additives many untested.

The average Western (non-European) diet uses only 20 foods.

The Italians select from 60 foods.

The Japanese have a saying that eating from less than 30 foods a day leads to ill health.

Ultra-processed (processed) foods (Nova classification) are industrial formulations with five ingredients, but usually many more. These ingredients include casein, lactose, whey, gluten and hydrogenated or inter-esterified oils.

Ultra-processed foods are also defined as "ready-to-eat" or "ready-to-heat" formulations made mostly from ingredients usually combined with additives.

Ultra-processed foods don't just include unhealthy things like fast food, soda, sugary soft drinks, chips, and hot dogs but ostensibly healthy or harmless foods like flavored yogurt, energy bars, baby formula, and cereal can also be, and mostly are, ultra-processed, as well as fast food, lunch meat, packaged bread, and most energy bars.

The best way to tell if something is ultra-processed is by scanning the nutrition label. If you see *a long list of ingredients you don't recognize*, chances are it's processed. And the scary part is that eating these foods—even just a couple times a week—could up your chances of dying prematurely, according to a new study.

One of my colleagues even goes so far as to say (and the more I think about it the more I like it), *"Just don't eat anything with a label on it"*.

Once upon a time they were a treat, but consumed habitually in excess, ultra-processed foods have become toxic.

Many of the packaged foods on our supermarket shelves are made "hyper-palatable" through chemical processing and "cosmetic" enhancement, such as the addition of colours, flavours and emulsifiers.

High in added sugar, fat and/or salt but with little, if any, nutritional value, they include confectionery snacks, fizzy drinks, cakes, sports drinks, many breakfast cereals, pastries, dehydrated vegetable soups and reconstituted meat and fish products.

Globally, these foods are believed to account for up to 60 per cent of daily energy intake (in Australia they account for about 35 per cent) and are already associated with obesity, high blood pressure, cholesterol and some cancers.

The Development of Processed Foods

World War 2 (WW2) boosted the research into nutrition and the processing of foods. Since then over 87,000 chemicals have been invented, many of which have found their way into our foods and the food chain. Most are untested and only investigated when there is some catastrophe.

Obesity was only "noticed" in the 1980s which means people were certainly getting fatter for some time prior. The current vogue in some medical quarters is to blame our genes or our gut microbiome *but these have not altered.*

The only thing that has altered is the food we eat.

I contend that the graph of this current overweigh-obesity epidemic would perfectly shadow the ingestion of processed foods - well close enough!

Processed, fast, pre-prepared, junk foods are full of these refined carbs and chemical additives and I think we simply cannot metabolise them.

Three studies suggest they are not good for you:

1. 105,159 volunteers completed three non-consecutive 24-hour dietary records in 2007 and were followed up to 2018. People who ate the most ultra-processed food had a 25 per cent increased risk of cardiovascular disease, compared with those who ate the least.

2. 19,899 Spanish students aged 20 and above completed food questionnaires from 1999. Those who ate the most ultra-processed food had a 62 per cent increased risk of death, compared with those who ate the least.

3. A June study from ANU (Australian National University) has linked processed foods with the development of Type 2 Diabetes (T2D) and cognitive decline, dementia and Alzheimer's.

PROCESSED POISON: Ready to Eat: Heat and Eat

The cumulative and cocktail effects of eating different processed foods "remain largely unknown". It is suggested that certain food additives may adversely affect cardiovascular health and that certain processing techniques may also be having a detrimental effect on our health.

The first study as to the effects of ultra-processed foods on health was published online February 11, 2019 in *JAMA Internal Medicine*. The Findings from this prospective study of a large French cohort suggest for the first time, that an increased proportion of ultra-processed foods in the diet is associated with a higher risk of overall mortality.

The University of Florida feels there is an association between processed food and the development of autism – but more research is needed.
A study of 105,159 French adults found that a 10 per cent increase in the amount of ultra-processed foods in the diet was associated with a significantly higher likelihood of ending up with cardiovascular disease, coronary heart disease and cerebrovascular disease (increases of 12, 13 and 11 per cent respectively). Those with a diet high in unprocessed or minimally processed foods, on the other hand, were significantly less likely to end up with any of these diseases.

Another study published found that participants on an ultra-processed diet gained weight, while participants on a minimally processed diet that contained the same amount of salts, fats and sugars and calories did not.

A second *BMJ* study, of nearly 20,000 Spanish adults over the course 10 years, found that eating more than four servings of ultra-processed foods a day (which is pretty easy when you consider that one serving of French fries is about 12 to 15 potato sticks) was associated with a 62 per cent increased risk of premature death by any cause, compared with less than two servings per day. Moreover, each additional serving of ultra-processed food was associated with a statistically significant 18 per cent higher hazard of all cause mortality.
All these increased as diets changed from eating home cooked fresh produce to eating ready-made foods.

It is estimated that, in the 1960s (before supermarkets became widespread), Australians had 600-800 foods available - very few ultra-processed. Now the average supermarket stocking more than 30,000 items - many ultra-processed. There are now over 87,000 "health" supplements.

Reformulating foods to lower the amount of salt, sugar or fat often meant increasing the amount of processing (such as adding artificial sweeteners to reduce total sugars in a product).

POISON: DO NOT EAT! – Well certainly minimise.

REFINED CARBS AND SIMPLE SUGARS (often called "added sugars")

Sugar: Table sugar/white sugar (aka sucrose; may be cane sugar or beet sugar)
Confectioner's sugar
Honey (Even though honey exists in nature and isn't refined, it is a pure sugar.)
Agave syrup

Corn syrup and high-fructose corn syrup
Brown sugar
Molasses
Maple syrup
Fructose
Brown rice syrup
Maltose
Glucose syrup
Tapioca syrup
Rice bran syrup
Malt syrup

Dextran
Sorghum
Treacle
Panela
Saccharose
Carob syrup
Dextrose, dextran, dextrin, maltodextrin
Fruit juice concentrates

Fruit Juices except for lemon/lime juice. Most fruit juices require special equipment to produce in significant quantities.

Instant/Refined Grains including instant hot cereals like instant oatmeal, white rice, polished rice, and instant rice

Refined Starches such as corn starch, potato starch, modified food starch–essentially any powdered ingredient with the word "starch" in it

All Kinds of Flour including wheat, oat, legume (pea and bean), rice, and corn flours. 100% stoneground, whole meal flours are less refined and not as unhealthy as other types of flours because they are not as finely ground and take longer to digest.

Soft Drinks / Sodas

Foods High in Refined Carbs and Added Sugars

All desserts except whole fruit
Ice cream, sherbet, frozen yogurt,
Most breads
Many crackers (100% stone-ground whole grain crackers are less refined)
Cookies; Cakes; Muffins; Pancakes; Waffles; Pies; Pastries; Candy; Chocolate (dark, milk and white). Baker's chocolate is unsweetened and is therefore an exception.
Breaded or battered foods
All doughs (phyllo, pie crust, etc)
Most cereals except for unsweetened, 100% whole grain cereals in which you can see the whole grains in their entirety with the naked eye (unsweetened muesli, rolled oats, or unsweetened puffed grain cereals are good examples)

Most pastas, noodles and couscous
Jelly (sugar-free varieties exist but it's much healthier to make your own with unsweetened gelatin and fresh fruit)
Jams and preserves
Bagels
Pretzels
Pizza (flour in the dough)
Puddings and custards
Corn chips
Caramel corn and kettle corn
Most granola bars, power bars, energy bars (unless sugar-free).
Rice wrappers
Tortillas (unless 100% stone-ground whole grain)
Most rice cakes and corn cakes (unless 100% whole grain)
Panko crumbs
Croutons

Fried vegetable snacks like green beans and carrot chips (usually contain added dextrin)
Ketchup
Honey mustard
Most barbecue sauces
Check labels on salsa, tomato sauces, salad dressings and other jarred/canned sauces for sugar/sweeteners
Sweetened yogurts and other sweetened dairy products
Honey-roasted nuts
Sweetened sodas
Chocolate milk (and other sweetened milks)
Condensed milk
Hot cocoa
Most milk substitutes (almond milk, soy milk, oat milk, etc) because they usually have sugar added–read label first
Sweet wines and liquors

Finally, it is absurd to deny ourselves some of these or to have a treat. The function here is to make you aware of just how we have come to accept many processed foods as being healthy such as corn chips, rice wrappers, fruits juices and pasta and to minimize or substitute fresh foods.

> **WE HUMANS CAN'T PROCESS PROCESSED FOODS**

GENERAL INFORMATION

Coffee and tea
The data on coffee are very good. Good as a substitute for sugary sodas
Most coffee data have been positive, even with high intake, though transient increases in blood pressure and anxiety can occur.

Milk
Milk consumption is an interesting adaptation in the human race since the advent of agriculture and lactase persistence in adults—meaning you can digest lactose into adulthood—has evolved six separate times over the past 6000 years. When suckling the human baby has an enzyme, *lactase,* which allows it to digest its mother's milk containing lactose. However, when weaned, many infants lose this lactase and now cannot digest milk containing lactose.

When humans moved out of the Rift Valley we were all black. Some went over to India and Australia and remained dark, others moved up toward Japan and became lighter while the third biggest migration moved to northern Europe and turned white. This pale skin allowed them to absorb more UVB from the sun to make vitamin D and absorb calcium, essential for bone, from milk and dairy but to be able to digest milk they had to retain their lactase. This is known as *lactase persistence.*

Clearly there's an evolutionary population advantage to it. Milk consumption may help explain why modern humans are so much taller than other hominids.

I have always claimed the Irish as 'genetically different' from the Celts or the English, Welsh and Scots as their skin seemed to me the worst of all for skin cancer. This, to me, is confirmed by the fact that lactase persistence is 100% in the Irish (and Finns).

People started avoiding dairy in part as reaction to the "China study," a large epidemiologic study that reported a correlation between dairy and cancer. But this is one of those cases where we take a correlational study and go crazy with it and its data have also been called into question.
Milk is reasonably nutrient dense and that is not pro- or anti-dairy.

Is Meat OK?
In the complete edition, The Medically Beneficial Diets, I detail how a Vegetarian Diet is "one of the healthiest". Be that as it may, no population has ever willingly adopted it because the tribe would have died out as humans need essential supplements, such as vitamin B12, which are not available from plants.

Furthermore, again as detailed elsewhere, humans have flat teeth (molars) that evolved to grind plants, but we also have pointed incisor and tearing "canine" teeth, which identify us as meat-eating animals.

One of the world's biggest studies the EPIC (European Prospective Investigation into Cancer and Nutrition) of more than half a million (521,000) participants but only some 448,568 from 10 different European countries followed for 12.7 years found that *"red meat posed no detectable risk as judged by all-cause mortality"*. *It did, however, find an association with processed meat.* Subsequent studies recommend we reduce meat to only twice a week

Most recently, the world's best coronary arteries yet studied were in the Tsimane people of the Bolivian Amazon have the lowest reported levels of vascular aging and the lowest prevalence of coronary atherosclerosis of any population yet studied and they eat meat - 14% of their diet. But you can bet it's lean, with no growth promoters or antibiotics and grass fed.

Meat has gained a bad reputation, but I think this is only because how it is prepared, especially searing with char marks, and much is fed an abnormal feed-lot diet which, in some countries also includes "growth promoters" aka steroids, and antibiotics. On top of this *we eat too much*. If you think about it our ancestors didn't get much meat. They had to chase a beast for days or weeks, so they were fit and lean but so was their kill! So they only ate lean meat occasionally...and it was grass fed or had eaten other meat eaters. Meat shortened the human gut, so we didn't have to eat all day like Herbivores and cooking it provided protein for our brains to grow bigger than any other animal. Meat was fundamental to human nutrition. It isn't now if you take the various supplements especially B12.

If you eat meat, make sure it's grass fed, lean and a small amount, not overcooked, only a couple of times a week. Processed meat such as bacon, ham and sausages are definitely bad for us and associated with cancer of the colon. I don't know if it were always thus and suspect the modern preservatives such as the nitrites may be carcinogenic. Poultry seems OK and so does pork again, organic is preferred.

However, it is to be emphasized that there's growing evidence that *high-protein food choices* do play a role in health—and that eating healthy protein sources like fish, chicken, beans, or nuts *in place of red meat* (especially processed red meat) can lower the risk of several diseases and premature death. A high ingestion of red meat increases the risks for cardiovascular disease, diabetes, cancer and osteoporosis.

How Much Red Meat is OK?
No one knows but a hell of a lot less than most people, eating the present Western Diet, consume. At the most I would suggest a steak no bigger than one's hand, twice a week and grass fed with no char on cooking.
Animal sources of protein tend to deliver all the amino acids we need.
Other protein sources, such as fruits, vegetables, grains, nuts and seeds lack one or more essential amino acids. Vegetarians need to be aware of this. People who don't eat meat, fish, poultry, eggs, or dairy products need to eat a variety of protein-containing foods each day in order to get all the amino acids needed to make new protein.

Are Eggs OK?
I would reduce them to two a week or one a day at most.

'Healthy' snacks fuelling rise in obesity among toddlers
Three-quarters of toddlers are being fed too much "healthy" snacks which are no better than sweets. Foods and drinks available to the under-threes found that the market for baby "finger food" – such as dried fruit and oat bars – is rapidly expanding. Processed dried fruit products were found to be the highest in sugar, prompting a warning that "these should not be marketed as suitable for children to eat between meals".

CHAPTER 4.
CARBOHYDRATES

Reduction improves metabolic syndrome independent of weight loss
Over the past five decades, carbohydrate consumption among Americans (and in most first world nations) have skyrocketed, and rates of metabolic syndrome along with it. The Metabolic Syndrome seems to be tied to insulin resistance, so avoiding insulin secretion (by limiting carb intake) makes sense. Low-carb diets have shown improvements in metabolic syndrome parameters, but those diets were *also* associated with weight loss. But a recent small but very well designed study organized the foods to have a total caloric content that would not lead to weight changes. This was not a weight-loss intervention; it was a pure dietary change intervention. It was to test if dietary carbohydrate intolerance (i.e., the inability to process carbohydrate in a healthy manner) rather than obesity per se is a fundamental feature of Metabolic Syndrome.

This study is regarded as the best so far to suggest that this relationship is not just driven by increases in weight but by the carbs themselves. A small but rigorous study appearing in *JCI Insight*. (2019;4(12):e128308, https://doi.org/10.1172/jci.insight.128308) suggests that a low-carb, high-fat diet improves the metabolic syndrome *even* when weight doesn't change.

Looking at the metabolic syndrome parameters, there was no significant change in waist circumference or blood pressure, but fasting glucose levels and triglycerides were significantly lower in the low-carb diet group, while HDL was higher. In fact, of the 16 individuals in the trial, nine no longer met criteria for metabolic syndrome after 4 weeks of the low-carb diet.

The Hi-Carb Diet was high in potatoes and a mix of whole and *processed grains* (My italics), with at least 5 servings of fruits and vegetables every day with fat cut out primarily from animal products (except for cheese). Unfortunately, they do not record just how much was processed. But, as can be seen from the following analysis the Low Carb diet (LC) consisted of only 45g of carbs compared with 420g for the High Carb (HC).

Table 1. Daily nutrient intake of controlled diets

Nutrient	HC	MC	LC
Energy (kcal)		2,950 (2035-3750)	
Protein (g)	144 (100-184)	146 (101-185)	150 (103-190)
Carbohydrate (g)	420 (290-534)	234 (161-297)	45 (31-58)
Fat (g)	77 (53-97)	159 (110-202)	242 (167-307)
Saturated fat (g)	40 (28-51)	70 (48-89)	100 (69-127)
Monounsaturated fat (g)	21 (15-27)	54 (37-69)	86 (59-110)
Polyunsaturated fat (g)	6 (5-8)	21 (14-26)	35 (24-45)
Cholesterol (mg)	334 (231-425)	503 (347-639)	1,015 (701-1291)
Cheese (g)	200 (138-255)	201 (139-256)	201 (139-256)
Calcium (mg)	2,151 (1484-2734)	2,229 (1537-2833)	2,177 (1502-2768)
Fiber (g)	25 (17-32)	20 (14-25)	14 (9-17)

This table is related to Figure 1. Values are mean (range). n = 16.

The conclusion is that a low carb diet would seem to be metabolically beneficial and, while this was not the point of this study, it can also be used to lose weight.

Inflammatory Diets

Participants who followed an inflammatory diet had almost twice the risk of developing colorectal cancer. An inflammatory diet is usually characterized by the consumption of refined carbohydrates, red and processed meat, and saturated or trans fats.

Processed Meat: "Generally speaking, a *processed* meat is one that has been salted, cured, smoked, fermented or undergone other processes to enhance flavor or improve preservation. Examples of processed meats include hot dogs (frankfurters), ham, sausage, corned beef, deli meats, and jerky.

Consuming 50 grams of processed meat a day—equivalent to just one hot dog—would raise the risk of getting colorectal cancer by 18 percent over a lifetime. Eating larger quantities raises cancer risk even more. Postmenopausal women who ate the most processed meat (an average of more than nine grams a day or the equivalent of about 1 and a quarter hot dogs a week) had a 21 percent higher risk of breast cancer than those who ate no processed meat.

It is not clear what component or components of processed meat are responsible for the association with cancer: While the exact culprit behind the association between processed meats and cancer is unclear, the association itself is convincing, especially for colorectal cancer, and the added sodium in these products has other clear negative health impacts. Cutting back on these foods, even if they say, "no added nitrates," is to berecommended.

Sodium: There is good evidence that consuming large quantities of foods preserved by salting is associated with increased risk of stomach, nasopharyngeal, and throat cancers. Deli meats (like pre-packaged turkey and ham slices) are one of the main sources.

Nitrates: Sodium nitrite and sodium nitrate (which naturally converts to sodium nitrite) are used as preservatives in processed meats because they prevent bacterial growth. Nitrates are also found naturally in a number of foods, including celery, beets, arugula, and other vegetables.

'No added nitrates' on processed meat products, usually means these products are manufactured using celery juice or other natural sources of nitrates but there is no evidence that the nitrates in celery juice act any differently in the body than nitrates added as food-grade chemicals. In fact, unlike food-grade sodium nitrate or nitrite, there is no federal regulation that limits how much celery juice can be added to a processed meat, so it is feasible to actually be consuming more nitrates with a processed meat that says, 'no added nitrates'. When consumed in vegetables, nitrates are safe, and may even have protective health effects such as improving blood flow. But in meats, nitrites can react during processing, cooking, and storage to form compounds called nitrosamines, which are classified as carcinogens. However, that the link between sodium nitrate and cancer risk is still unclear.

Cooking: There is not enough data to prove that the way meat is cooked affects cancer risk, but it is known that cooking meat (processed or unprocessed) at high temperatures or in direct contact with heat (such as grilling or pan-frying) produces more carcinogenic chemicals than lower-heat, indirect methods like roasting or stewing.

BOOK 2

SUCCESSFUL AGING

From childhood

Staying
- **fit**
  - **functioning**
  - **financial**

Avoiding declines in capacity and health
The Quality of Life and Death

FROM WOMB TO TOMB

Successful ageing starts in the womb.

We are at our healthiest aged 11 years. Many people tacitly accept "growing old", getting fat, becoming more sedentary and more dependent on others. Some do this, years, even decades, before others.

This need not be.

By preventing illnesses, eating correctly and keeping fit while adopting a healthy lifestyle, there is now no reason why we should not live into our 90s, fit, functioning, independent with all our marbles.

But we are not aware of these changes which only first become apparent in our 40s unless, as here, we are made aware of these changes.

Our early lifestyles and diet cause the problems that kill or disable us prematurely. The earlier we can start to look after ourselves the better – but it's never too late.

I think every 17 year-old should read this when they leave school or even earlier. But parents should inculcate these preventive measures to give their kids the best chance of a healthy life and it is really critical to institute these recommendations in our 40s.

It would seem the ambition of most to retire aged around 60 years of age but, as you will see, such people die early.

Overall our aim should be to have a job or interests and certainly not become aimless and lonely with no purpose(s). But we are living longer than Governments can afford to support us so financial security it imperative which, for those self-employed, too often comes as a shock they have not planned for.

Most illnesses are preventable and normal age changes minimized, but you have to know what to do…no matter how young or how old you are e.g. Most of us don't know that from the age of 30 years we lose 1% of muscle mass every year but moderate correct exercise minimizes this and keeps us mobile.

Research has pointed out that age changes are mostly attributable to inactivity. Optimum ageing necessitates exercise. Inevitably, our bodies will experience declines with age, but staying physically active can buy extra years of function compared to sedentary people.

CHAPTER 1.
WHAT IS SUCCESSFUL AGING

Concepts: What do people regard as 'successful':
1. Something beyond health & longevity: The 'good life' in late life - the capacity to function across all of life's parameters
2. The Quality of Life and Death
3. Aging that is better than 'usual aging' - avoidance of declines in capacity & health

Changing Concepts
The criteria for Successful Aging increase as people live longer and society becomes more complex and so do expectations and it is a *changing concept*. It is important to consider the broader concerns of the individual, but the fundamental basis is having the ability, facilities and money to enjoy a good, contented life and this requires some forward planning of not just health but all social parameters. If we live longer, then how will we mentally cope with age, and at a more practical level, will we have enough money and where will we end up, also comes into play. Successful aging includes cognitive, physical, social, spiritual, emotional & economic parameters and the capacity to cope with change.

Younger Concepts
It strikes me that the above concepts are those of people who 'suddenly' realise they are getting old and have to face facts. As stated, I think Successful Aging starts in the womb and we must provide the best and educate our kids as to life-long healthy behaviours and lifestyles.

Junk food, poor diet, sugary drinks, poor dental care, lack of exercise, too much screen time and a polluted environment are childhood harbingers of a shortened lifespan and premature avoidable illnesses. As teenagers smoking and drugs must be prevented, and booze controlled.

Western civilisation, however, is geared and motivated against almost every aspect of starting life so as to successfully age: Junk food is the standard diet for impoverished students or apprentice tradesmen, smoking was a rite of passage, the mobile phone is a fixture, sport now 'professional' and not there for fun, cars belch out micro-particles and the Friday night binge another rite of passage along with sunbaking and desire for a tan.

The reaction against this has been to become obsessional by becoming a vegan and a gym junkie which are as anti-social and disruptive as being glued to a mobile phone screen.

But, until we encounter some health shock or hit 40, we are bullet proof with no tomorrow.

Early Measures: Parental Responsibility
While Successful Aging should being in utero, kids and teenagers oblivious to heath issues and most of us until we are 30 or 40 giving no real thought as to aging, let alone 'successfully', it therefore *depends on parenting to inculcate good nutrition and behaviours* which have been already documented in Books 1 and 3 However, while most of the following issues are from the aspect of older persons, the lists of the Age Changes in the **Actual Practical Impediments and Actual Medical Causative Conditions** in Chapter 2, start at 18 years of age and that, hopefully, is when some good lifestyle and preventive habits may be assumed.

The alarming degradation is just every-day functions from age 18, as these lists document, should be, hopefully, enough to make most of us to think and adopt the best lifestyles.

Main Constituents of Successful Aging
The increase in life expectancy has added to defining what is successful aging and who should define it, not the least of which should be the elderly themselves, as well as medical experts.

As noted, these concepts are now for the elderly whereas it is obvious these issues should be addressed in childhood.

Main Theoretical constituents
A very complete survey and review consulted provides the following.
- Life expectancy
- Life satisfaction and well-being (includes happiness and contentment)
- Mental and psychological health, cognitive function
- Personal growth, learning new things
- Physical health and functioning, independent functioning
- Psychological characteristics and resources including perceived autonomy, control, independence, adaptability, coping, self-esteem, positive outlook, goals, sense of self
- Social, community, leisure activities, integration and participation
- Social networks, support, participation, activity
- People are more successful in taking up healthy habits if their partner makes positive changes

- Mortality was lower in people who felt younger (14%) than those who felt their actual age (19%) or older (25%). After adjustment for covariates (e.g., age, ethnicity, sex), feeling older than chronological age was a significant independent predictor of mortality. A relationship existed between self-perceived age and cardiovascular death but not cancer death.
- A study of 9,050 English people with an average age of 65 found that the people with the greatest wellbeing, with a purpose and sense of meaning, conferring a sense of control, feeling activities were worthwhile with sense of purpose in life, were 30% less likely to die during the average eight-and-a-half-year follow-up period than those with the least wellbeing.
- Appetite is generally regarded as one of the most important indicators of health while a poor appetite may be a valuable early indicator of incipient nutritionally related disorders and disease, and of premature mortality.

Three main domains
1. *Medical*: avoidance of disease and disability (Missing Keys Book 3)
2. *Psychosocial*: mental state (life satisfaction, acceptance of death)
3. *Lay*: Elderly peoples' own views

1. *Medical* focus on:
   - the absence of chronic disease and of risk factors for disease
   - good health
   - high levels of independent physical functioning
   - performance, mobility
   - cognitive functioning.

However, this fails to address the implications of the fact that a disease-free older age is unrealistic for most people.

2. Psychosocial
Emphasize life satisfaction, social participation and functioning, and psychological resources, including personal growth.

3. Lay
Aging people's own concerns:
1. Psychological factors
2. Social roles and activities
3. Finances
4. Social relationships
5. Neighbourhood

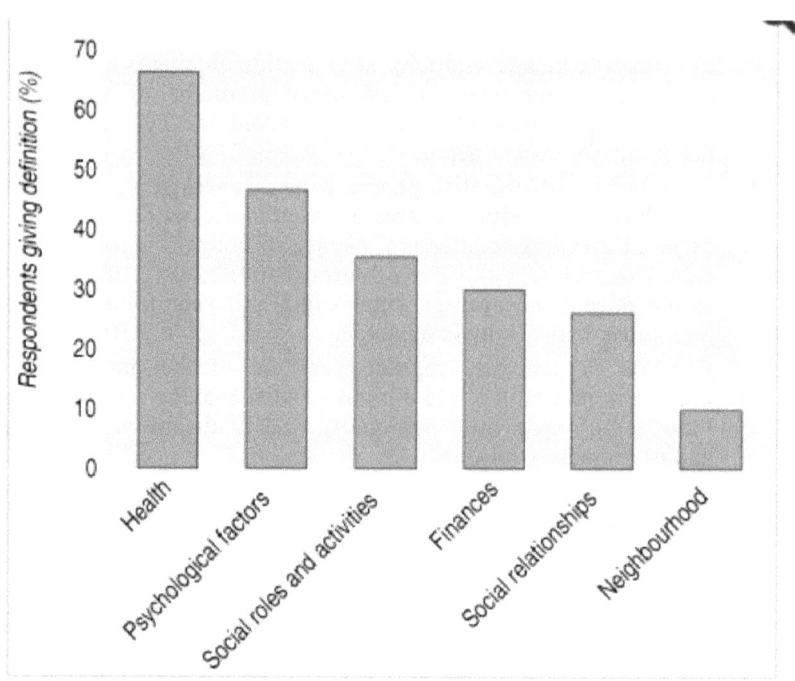

Ageing Concerns

Health
It is noteworthy that health far outstrips all other concerns in this survey of ageing people.

Ageing People's Greatest Health Concerns
For most people health is their greatest concern growing old and the illnesses that they are most concerned about are according to one TV survey are:

1. Dementia 66%
2. Cancer 40%
3. Heart D 30%
4. Cholesterol 29%
5. Diabetes 25%
6. 5-day 25%
7. Exercise 24%
8. Sugar 20%

Summary
Successful Aging means living our natural maximum lifespan while maintaining our Quality of Life rather than simply aiming to support elderly people with chronic conditions.

CHAPTER 2.
AGE CHANGES: WHAT TO EXPECT (and AVOID)

Aging represents the accumulation of changes in a human being over time, encompassing physical, psychological, and social changes. Most are insidious, and we are unaware when these inexorable changes of age start and progress.

It is necessary to have a firm, achievable goal as to how we want to, and should, age. To that end, I repeat the Live Longest definition of Quality of Life:

Live Longest Definition
Optimization of present health and fitness: to minimize any illnesses and disabilities; to stay mentally alert, active, healthy, independent and socially integrated, with the capacity to cope with change; for the whole of our predicted lifespan with respect to personal, social, spiritual, emotional and economic goals (financial security) and restrictions.

While this is a mouthful, it covers all areas and contingencies, many of which we don't consider when we are young—such as being able to remain independent with enough money to do so.

This, in effect, is what to strive for.

We are at our healthiest aged 11 years. Until age 20 or so, we need food to grow tall and lay down muscle and bone but not fat. However, when we reach the age of 20 years, age changes start and now and we stop growing and rather than muscle and bone, fat is laid down and it is more difficult to keep our figure or lose weight, and while we are aware of this change there are other more insidious changes happening.

- Over this time, from aged 18 years to over 65
- Hearing of normal conversation becomes 11 times worse
- Climbing stairs becomes 15 times worse
- Lifting 10 lb or 5 kg 10 times harder
- Getting in and out of bed 12 times more difficult
- And on and on, as listed on the next pages.

Study the next two pages as to the changes for the three age groups. They can be startlingly depressing, but their great feature is that they identify where we age, such that we can address and minimize these changes. On the next page are the causes of disabilities which while they are not actual causes of age changes can accelerate them and hence, we should avoid them (Book 1).

If you know what you are likely to encounter you can avoid, prevent or minimise them.

> **If you know what you are likely to encounter you can avoid, prevent or minimize them.**

Live Longest Compendium   63

ACTUAL PRACTICAL IMPEDIMENTS:

Most are unaware of these changes and how they progress to impact on our lives:

	% 18 - 44	% 45 - 64	→% 65 yrs
Difficulty specified functions	6.3	19.4	47.5
Seeing words/letters in newsprint	1.3	3.8	→
Hearing normal conversation	1.1	3.6	11.2
Having speech understood	0.8	1.1	2.1
Walking three city blocks	2.9	11.3	31.7
Climbing a flight of stairs	2.8	11.4	30.2
Grasping objects	1.0	4.2	8.2
Lifting/Carrying 10 lbs	2.3	7.8	21.8
Difficulty daily living activities	1.0	4.1	12.5
Getting around inside home	0.4	1.8	6.4
Getting in/out of bed/chair	0.6	2.7	7.5
Bathing	0.6	2.2	7.9
Dressing	0.5	1.7	5.3
Eating	0.2	0.6	2.1
Toileting	0.3	1.0	3.6
Difficulty instrumental daily activities	2.2	6.0	19.1
Getting around outside of home	1.1	3.8	13.7
Taking care of money and bills	1.1	1.7	7.4
Preparing meals	0.8	1.8	8.0
Doing light housework	0.9	3.2	9.9
Managing prescriptions	0.7	1.6	6.2
Using the telephone	0.4	0.8	4.6
Reporting of selected impairments	5.6	6.9	8.1
A learning disability	2.2	1.3	0.6
Mental retardation	0.7	0.4	0.3
Other developmental disability	0.4	0.2	0.1
Alzheimer's/Dementia/Senility	o.3	0.6	3.8
Other mental/emotional disability	3.5	5.6	5.6
Use of assistive aid	1.0	4.6	19.2
Wheelchair	0.4	1.3	5.2
Cane, crutches, or walker	0.8	4.2	17.9
Limitation to work around the house	3.5	10.7	20.3
Limitation to work at a job or business	4.5	11.3	

Estimated number* and percentage of civilian noninstitutionalized adults aged ≥18 years with self-reported disabilities, by age group --- United States, 2005

ACTUAL MEDICAL CAUSATIVE CONDITIONS

Main cause of disability among U.S. adults aged ≥18 years with self-reported disabilities.

Conditions	Total %	Men %	Women %
Arthritis or rheumatism	19.0	11.5	24.3
Back or spine problems	16.8	16.9	16.8
Heart trouble	6.6	8.4	5.4
Lung or respiratory problem	4.9	4.9	4.9
Mental or emotional problem	4.9	5.2	4.6
Diabetes	4.5	4.8	4.2
Deafness or hearing problem	4.2	6.8	2.4
Stiffness or deformity of limbs/	3.6	3.6	3.7
Blindness or vision problem	3.2	3.9	2.8
Stroke	2.4	3.1	1.9
Cancer	2.2	2.4	2.1
Broken bone/fracture	2.1	1.9	2.3
High blood pressure	1.9	1.6	2.1
Mental retardation	1.5	1.7	1.3
Senility/Dementia/Alzheimer's	1.2	1.0	1.3
Head or spinal cord injury	1.1	1.5	0.9
Learning disability	1.1	1.6	0.7
Kidney problems	0.9	1.2	0.7
Stomach/Digestive problems	0.8	0.7	0.8
Paralysis of any kind	0.6	0.7	0.5
Epilepsy	0.6	0.6	0.6
Hernia or rupture	0.5	0.6	0.5
Cerebral palsy	0.5	0.8	0.3
Missing limbs/extremities	0.5	0.8	0.2
Alcohol or drug problem	0.4	0.8	0.2
Tumor/Cyst/Growth	0.3	0.2	0.3
Thyroid problems	0.2	0.1	0.3
AIDS or AIDS-related	0.2	0.2	0.2
Speech disorder	0.2	0.1	0.2
Other	12.9	12.1	13.5
Total*	100.0	100.0	100.0

USA OVERALL CAUSES OF DISABILITY IN MEN

Disability	% Affected
Back or spinal problems	16.9
Arthritis or Rheumatism	11.5
Heart trouble	8.4
Deafness or impeded hearing	6.6
Mental or emotional problems	5.2
Lung or respiratory problems	4.9
Diabetes	4.8
Vision problems or blindness	3.9
Stiffness or deformity of limbs	3.6
Stroke	3.1
Cancer	2.4
Fractures – broken bones	1.9

FURTHER AGE CHANGES

The five senses: All incur sensory loss with age,

1. Vision
2. Touch
3. Smell
4. Taste
5. Hearing

Eyesight:

- People over 35 years of age are at risk for lens shrinkage and developing presbyopia (having to push the paper away to read) and most people benefit from reading glasses by age 45–50. The cause is lens hardening, a process which may be sped up by higher temperatures and exposure
- Cataracts: light reaching 60 yr. retina is one third that at 20yrs. Cataracts are evident by age 80, and more than half of all Americans have cataract surgery. Queensland, the Sun Belt-sun cancer capital of the world, has four times more. Reduced vision limits non-verbal communication, isolation possible depression.
- Macular Degeneration causes vision loss and increases with age, affecting nearly 12% of those above the age of 80. This degeneration is from systemic changes in the circulation of waste products and growth of abnormal vessels around retina.
- Age-related macular degeneration (AMD) is a condition in which the eye's macula, responsible for our sharpest vision, begins to thin and break down, causing vision loss. If left untreated may lead to blindness. There is no surefire way to prevent AMD. However,
    1. Smoking can speed up AMD damage. If you smoke, quit.
    2. Sunlight is thought to possibly promote AMD. Protect your eyes from the sun by wearing sunglasses and broad-brimmed hats.
    3. Research also suggests that certain nutrients help prevent macular degeneration. One supplement that may work combines a mixture of (all) three light-absorbing compounds; *lutein, zeaxanthin and meso-zeaxanthin.* However, many researchers believe that simply eating a diet rich in fresh fruits and dark-green leafy vegetables, such as spinach, collard greens, kale, rich in lutein and zeaxanthin, keys for eye health, should be enough.
    4. If you have intermediate or advanced dry AMD, or any stage of the "wet" form, ask your doctor about any new medications.

Hearing Loss:
Occurs in one third of people between 65 and 74 and half of those older than 75. Hearing loss at high-frequency above 20 kHz becomes apparent in teenagers

Taste:
Diminishes with age leading to the use of more salt and spices

Hair:
Loss of hair pigment. Hair turns grey. Pattern hair loss by the age of 50 affects about half of males and a quarter of females

Skin:
- Wrinkles mainly due to photo aging, particularly sun-exposed areas
- Increased fragility of skin and blood vessels
- Lipofuscin subcutaneous deposition (yellowish deposits)
- Reduced sweat gland efficiency (heat exhaustion / stroke)
- Poor healing of connective tissue

Bones and Joints:
- Osteoporosis, loss of height, fractures
- Osteoarthritis rises in the 60–64 age cohort, to 53%. Of which 20% report disabling
- Spinal lordosis – (tips head forward causing choking)
- Neglected feet
- Back pain can't bend

Blood Vessels:
- Atherosclerosis – narrowing of the arteries is classified as an aging disease. It leads to cardiovascular disease (for example hypertension, stroke and heart attack) which globally is the most common cause of death

Fitness:
- Reduced exercise capacity
- Slower walking speed
- Greater intra-abdominal fat, glucose intolerance, dyslipidemia
- Female fertility peaks in the mid-20s and declines
- Menopause typically occurs between 49 and 52 years of age
- Altered immune status - susceptible to infections and illness
- Reduced living standards / Diminished Quality of Life (QOL)

Nervous System: Less sensitivity to nerve stimulus
- Cognitive decline begins in the mid-20s
- Memory impairment
- Dementia becomes more common with age.
  - About 3% of people between the ages of 65 and 74,
  - 19% between 75 and 84, and
  - nearly half of those over 85 years

SARCOPENIA – Muscle loss with age

Needs special attention because it is insidious but, if we lose our strength, we lose mobility and it's then a rapid deteriorating, downwards spiral.

Frailty: Defined as loss of muscle mass and mobility, affects 25% of those over 85.

Even healthy people lose strength @ 1-2% pa and power @ 3-4%pa
- After age 30   =   2 – 3 %   pa
- After age 60   =   10%   pa
- 65 – 70 yrs.   =   13 to 24%   pa
- After 80   =   50%
- i.e. there is a loss of some 35% to 40% of muscle between ages 20 to 80 years
- Most rapid loss for men is between 40 and 60 years and for women after 60
- 30 yr olds need only 50 - 60% quadriceps to rise from sitting: 90 yr olds need 95%
- 50% women, 15% men 70–74yrs are too weak to mount 30 cm step without a handrail
- Maximum Oxygen Uptake Rate (VO2 max) defines endurance exercise capacity
- A decrease in muscle mass decreases the VO2 max at the rate of 1% per annum
- This is reflected in a decreased aerobic capacity
- Resistance training increases VO2 max. It's never too late 55-75 yr olds have shown
- Inactivity affects the muscular strength in young and older men equally

Falls
Over 30% of people > 65 yrs fall each year. The risk increases each year
- * Osteoporosis – most important

Best prevention:
- * Awareness / admission..
- * Muscle strengthening
- * Balance retraining. No standing on chairs after age 60
- * Walking Risk avoidance. Get assistance

Hand Grip Strength
A simple grip strength test may predict metabolic disorders in middle or older age.

Low normal grip strength was greatly associated with both cardio-metabolic diseases and physical disabilities in middle age to older adults, both men and women.

This may sound too simplistic but, if you think about it, the strength in our hands, our most used physical attribute, would well and truly reflect our overall physical fitness.

FURTHER CHANGES

Diseases of Affluence: We live in an era of unprecedented affluence with resulting diseases: Obesity, Hypertension, Heart Attacks, Strokes, Diabetes 2, Hyperlipidaemia (cholesterol / triglycerides), Blood pressure, Stress / depression, Skin cancer

Weight Gain - The Middle-Aged Spread
- There is both an absolute gain in weight, and also a relative percentage increase in fat between 40 and 50 years of age from 28% to 35% with central adiposity.

Living Standards Fall with Age: Where's the Money Gone?
Living standards will be squeezed by 27% = $6,500 pa over the next 40 years. That is probably more like $10,000 pa today and then indexed.

Diseases of Changed Circumstances or Poverty in Affluent Societies
While affluence has seen food become available, good, healthy nutritious foods, especially fruit, have become expensive such that people forced to economize now prefer cheaper processed foods which contribute to the epidemic of obesity and its sequelae. Junk-Processed Food is three times cheaper than healthy food.

External Appearance vs. Internal
If someone is proud enough to keep fit, lean and with beautiful skin it is my experience his or her whole body reflects this high standard. Good looks, good coronary arteries, good brain.

Modifiable lifestyle characteristics
- physical inactivity
- obesity
- tobacco use

These are major causes of disability often from a primary disabling condition.

Chances of becoming disabled: >40% if overweight and smoking

A typical female, age 35, 5'4", 125 pounds, non-smoker, works mostly an office job, with some outdoor physical responsibilities, and who leads a healthy lifestyle has the following risks:
- A 24% chance of becoming disabled for 3 months or longer during her working career,
- a 38% chance that the disability would last 5 years or longer and with the average disability for someone like her lasting 82 months.

If this same person used tobacco and weighed 160 pounds,
- risk would increase to a 41% chance of becoming disabled for 3 months or longer.

A typical male, age 35, 5'10", 170 pounds, non-smoker, who works an office job, with some outdoor physical responsibilities, and who leads a healthy lifestyle has the following risks:
- A 21% chance of becoming disabled for 3 months or longer in his working career
- a 38% chance that the disability would last 5 years or longer and with the average disability for someone like him lasting 82 months.

If this same person used tobacco and weighed 210 pounds,
- the risk would increase to a 45% chance of becoming disabled for 3 months (+)

Rates of non-fatal diseases and injuries are declining more slowly than death rates.

Just one in 20 people worldwide (4.3%) had no health problems in 2013.

The recent improvement in statistics helps identify what are cumbersomely labeled "Non-Fatal Burdens of Disease" (NFBD). I think we can just call them "Burdens" as it's hard to conceive a burden if we are dead. These new statistics allow construction of a logical, systematic and focused preventive or minimization plan.

It would seem all of us are destined to be burdened in some way in our final years. The aim is to make this as short as possible Compression of Morbidity: A reduction in the proportion of years spent with disability or ill health or *"healthy longer, sicker shorter"*

The Baby Boomer generation, which is now reaching old age, is not seeing improvements in health similar to the older groups that went before them. Only for people aged 65 and older was there this compression of morbidity. However, by contrast, the latest study shows that the increase in life expectancy in the past two decades has been accompanied by an even greater increase in life years free of disability, which is the main aim of this game - Compression of Morbidity (Sicker shorter, healthier longer).

Clearly, there is a need to maintain health and reduce disability at younger ages to have meaningful compression of morbidity across the age ranges.

Multiple Chronic Conditions (MCC)– Disabilities
Approximately 25% of U.S. adults have diagnoses of MCC. Data from the 2014 National Health Interview Survey (NHIS) were used to estimate prevalence of MCC (defined as two or more of 10 diagnosed chronic conditions).

CHAPTER 3.
SUCCESSFUL vs. ANTI-AGING

Anti-aging is trying to look younger or hopefully delay the changes of age. **Successful Aging** is the effective coping with, optimizing and minimization of age changes.

The corollary is Unsuccessful Aging: The unthinking, passive acceptance of age changes, consequent accelerated aging, increasing sedentary behaviour and the Diseases of Affluence.

Anti and Successful Aging are not mutually exclusive: Obviously people, determined to look young, have a vested interest in optimizing their health and welfare and may well incorporate Successful Aging but cosmetically looking younger is not essential for Successful Aging.

Statement by 51 Pre-eminent Scientists

* *"Since recorded history individuals have been, and are continuing to be, victimized by promises of extended youth or increased longevity by using unproven methods that allegedly slow, stop or reverse aging.*

* *There are no lifestyle changes, surgical procedures, vitamins, antioxidants, hormones or genetic engineering available today that do so.*

* *What medical science can tell us is that because age and death are not programmed into our genes, health and fitness can be enhanced at any age, primarily through avoidance of behaviour (such as smoking, excess alcohol, excess sun & obesity) that accelerate aging and adopt behaviours (such as exercise & a healthy diet) that give advantage to a physiology that is inherently modifiable".*

The foundations of Anti-aging, as well as Successful Aging, are best achieved by not abusing ourselves with High-Risk Behaviours and an evidenced healthy lifestyle – mainly good nutrition and exercise (Books 1, 3, 4 and 5).

CHAPTER 4.
LONGEVITY & LIFE EXPECTANCY

Successful Aging, above all, means optimising our health and compression of morbidity - "healthy longer, shorter ill".

Definition: Longevity is *not dying prematurely.*

Healthy Life Expectancy
A study in the *Lancet* shows that across the developed world life expectancies continue to climb, pushing above 90 for the first time

- Healthy Life Expectancy is increasing at a faster rate than Total Life Expectancy suggesting that reductions in mortality are accompanied by reductions in disability.
- People living in the poorest areas die younger (by 6 years) and also spend twice as many years in poor health

Rank	Country ESTIMATED LIFE EXPECTANCY 2017	Years
1.	Monaco	89.42
2.	Japan	85.26
3.	Singapore	85.21
4.	Macau	84.55
5.	San Marino	83.34
6.	Andorra	82.85
7.	Guernsey	82.61
8.	Hong Kong	82.52
9.	Australia	82.31
10.	Italy	82.28

Future Life Expectancy 2030
The UK Medical Research Council and US Environmental Protection Agency funded a study published in February 2017 of "Future life expectancy in 35 industrialized countries" and it concluded by 2030 Life Expectancy is projected to increase in all countries studied with the greatest improvements for women being South Korea, France and Spain replacing Japan. While for men the order will be South Korea, Australia, Switzerland then Canada.

Women Live Longer Than Men
Humans are the only species in which one sex lives longer than the other which is considered a survival advantage and one of the most robust features of human biology.

But the female advantage has some drawbacks in that for all their robustness relative to men in terms of survival, women on average appear to be in poorer health than men through adult life. This higher prevalence of physical limitations in later life is seen not only in Western societies. However, that the gap is narrowing as women join the workforce, smoke and drink more. The female life expectancy advantage over men is likely to shrink by 2030.

REALISTIC EXPECTATIONS

Life expectancy varies from country to country, even from suburb to suburb, and conclusions can be drawn by examination of these: The higher the standard of living, health system and medical care the longer the lives. This means a clean water supply, good sewerage systems, good hygiene and good (nutritional), adequate food.

While the USA comes in at 53rd for overall life expectancy it has an overwhelming 50 people in the top 100 verified longest living people, Japan has 19, the UK has eight and France six while the countries with the longest overall life expectancy don't have anyone in the Top 100 except Spain with three, Italy with two and Australia with one. One conclusion it would seem is that the overall average in the USA is poor because the lower end of its society is not as medically well cared for compared with the welfare state of the UK, but its upper rich-end people accesses the best medical care and conditions in the world.

There are pockets of civilization, called the Blue Zones, where people live longer than their national average. Sardinians live longer than most Italians, Okinawans live longer than most Japanese, isolated communities in Greece or tribes in Central America live far longer than their national average.

While there are advances being made and to be made, the present lifespan we should aim for and reasonably expect is our mid-80s.

Longevity: Genes or Lifestyle
The New England Study into Centenarians suggests that centenarians beget centenarians. In other words, genetics is a factor in longevity, but the estimates vary from 6% to 30%. In any event, to live longer, at least

> 70% is due to modifiable factors. Studies of longer living communities in Okinawa, Costa Rica, Sicily and elsewhere, suggest that life span can be increased by up to 8 years (in addition to any genetic or gender advantages) through, obviously good, lifestyle practices. We may not be able to choose our parents (or our gender) but we can certainly choose to minimize the risks we take with our health which is lifelong and begins early (sun damage to our skin, then smoking, would be obvious examples).

However, not only do the children of centenarians live longer but so do their siblings, which suggests genes play a larger role in exceptional old age.

Exceptional Longevity in Men: Modifiable Factors to Age 90 Years
Of 970 men (41%) who survived to at least age 90 years:

- Smoking was associated with increased risk of mortality before age 90 years. Similar associations were observed with diabetes, obesity and hypertension.
- Regular exercise was associated with a nearly 30% lower mortality risk.
- The probability of a 90-year life span at age 70 years was 54% in the absence of smoking, diabetes, obesity, hypertension, or sedentary lifestyle.
- It ranged from 36% to 22% with 2 adverse factors and was negligible (4%) with 5.
- Compared with non-survivors, men with exceptional longevity had a healthier lifestyle (67% vs. 53% had 1 adverse factor), had a lower incidence of chronic diseases, and were 3 to 5 years older at disease onset.
- They had a better late-life physical function and mental well-being.
- More than 68% (vs. 45%) rated their late-life health as excellent or very good, andless than 8% (vs. 22%) reported fair or poor health.

Weight, Mortality, Years of Healthy Life & Active Life Expectancy in Older
Healthy women who have normal weight at age 65 have a life expectancy of 22.1 years

Living to 100: Lifestyle advice for would-be centenarians

For the past 50 years, researchers have followed the health of 855 men born in 1913. Now that the study is being wrapped up, it turns out that ten of the subjects lived to 100 and conclusions can be drawn about the secrets of their longevity. Various surveys at the age of 54, 60, 65, 75, 80 and 100 permitted the researchers to consider the factors that appear to promote longevity. A total of 27% of the original group lived to the age of 80 and 13% to 90. 1.1% of the subjects made it to their 100th birthday.

- 42% of deaths after the age of 80 were due to cardiovascular disease
- 20% to infectious diseases
- 8% to stroke, 8% to cancer
- 6% to pneumonia
- 16% to other causes
- 23% of the over-80 group was diagnosed with some type of dementia.

Recommendations for people who aspire to centenarianism is to

- refrain from smoking,
- maintain healthy cholesterol levels and
- confine themselves to four cups of coffee a day.
- It also helps if you paid a high rent for a flat or owning a house at age 50 (indicating good socio-economic standard),
- enjoy robust working capacity at a bicycle test when you are 54
- and have a mother who lived for a long time. A correlation with maternal but not paternal longevity found that this "genetic factor" weaker than other factors.

The Roles of Disability and Morbidity in Survival to Exceptional Old Age

Although it is commonly held that survival to age 100 years entails markedly delaying or escaping age-related morbidities, calling on data from the New England Centenarian Study, nearly one-third of centenarians have age-related morbidities for 15 or more years. Yet, as previously observed, many centenarians compress disability toward the end of their lives. Therefore, it has been hypothesized that for some centenarians, compression of disability rather than morbidity is a key feature for survival to old age. This conforms my Live Longest recommendations in Book 3 to "Get it seen, Get it diagnosed. Get it better".

Lifestyle High-Risk Behaviours to Be Addressed:

    Tobacco – Cigarette Smoking
    Processed foods
    Eating habits – processed and junk foods – lack of fruit/vegetables
    Exercise patterns – physical inactivity
    High blood pressure
    Drinking habits – alcohol harm
    Weight – overweight/underweight
    High LDL
    Driving style
    Hobbies – high-risk - head trauma from sport
    Occupations – high risk
    Pesticides, industrial-workplace toxins (nail salons)
    Diesel fumes / Air pollution
    Unsafe sex
    Illicit drugs
    Lack of vaccinations
    Hygiene
    Loud music, noise
    Glare
    Sunburn

The LONGEST LIVING PEOPLE

As of 8 April 2019, the oldest known living person is Kane Tanaka of Japan, aged 116 years, 96 days. The oldest known living man is Gustav Gerneth of Germany, aged 113 years, 175 days. The world's oldest authenticated person was Jeanne Louise Calment, who lived in France and ostensibly reached the age of 122 years (died 1997) but it now seems there is some doubt as to the veracity of this.

It would seem that around 120 years is, at present, as long as the human can live. There is, however, much research to extend this.

The Seven Population Groups Who Live Longest: The Blue Zones

The Blue Zones was coined to identify a geographic area where people live longer The reasons for longevity in the Blue Zones are thought to be due to their

1. 'Primitive' diet of fresh foods and vegetables
2. Reduced amount of meat and saturated / trans fats
3. Age accepted as a normal progression where respect, physical work and activity is pursued and continued
4. Eating less / keeping lean
5. Family focus,
6. Social integration and activity
7. Less smoking

Buettner in his book provide a list of nine recommendations:

1. Moderate, regular physical activity.
2. Life purpose.
3. Stress reduction.
4. Moderate calories intake.
5. Plant-based diet.
6. Moderate alcohol intake
7. Engagement in spirituality or religion.
8. Engagement in family life.
9. Engagement in social life.

These are the essential basics and form part of all recommendations. However, there is now a great deal more evidence and sophistication to be recommended.

These basic groups (with the exception of the Adventists of California and Mormons) are incorporating the lifestyle, diet and conditions, which have evolved to be their way of life. Basically they are peasant communities who grow their own produce and are physically active. They have, or had, no options.

We do. And, sadly, these Blue Zones community-supported lifestyles, and diets will now be exposed to the now universal commercial pressures.

We have to combat these potentially damaging and life shortening intrusions endemic in our society, such as processed foods and sedentary lifestyles, and we can only do this by identifying what may be bad for us and what illnesses we may avoid.

Blue Zone Longevity Conclusions:

- Active, lean and fit
- No retirement
- No overeating. Okinawans stop when they feel 80% full
- 'Eat less and live longer'.
- No empty calories: Low calorie, high nutrition food.
- Fresh local produce in season
- Mostly vegetarian
- Good carbohydrates – vegetables, fruit and grains
- Protein – mostly from plants – beans, peas, whole grains, seeds nuts.
- No processed foods
- Low in fats from natural sources – nuts, seeds, fish – none from bottles, no margarine or butter
- Socially engaged, integrated, active and supported,
- Age is respected,
- Adversity faced and coped with
- Happiness and being content with one's lot is commonplace

New forecasts on life expectancy cast doubt on whether Australians will continue to live longer and healthier lives. As the rising obesity and high rates of road accident death and suicide among young people are predicted to overwhelm future gains in medical science that should allow Australians to live even longer. This has compelled the Australian Bureau of Statistics to wind back long-term life expectancy projections, the first time the index has dipped — an unprecedented turnaround in life expectancy.

The long-running gains in life expectancy began in the 1970s and accelerated in the 80s and 1990s, fuelled by public health measures such as anti-smoking campaigns, good diet promotion and efforts to reduce the road toll. These, plus advances in medicine, brought a dramatic reduction in premature deaths, particularly due to cardiovascular disease.

In about 2010, however, that long-term decline in cardiovascular mortality stopped in Australia, while in the US, Britain and Canada, cardiovascular mortality rates had started to rise again. Rising rates of obesity are a major contributor, along with stubborn rates of smoking. Separately, there has been a concerning rise in youth suicide in recent years and difficulty reducing the road toll.

WHY WE AGE

The Two Aging Processes: Humans age in two different ways.

1.) Normal aging is the result of cellular processes. This process occurs naturally, without the influence of disease, and currently limits the maximum lifespan to around 120 years.

2.) Pathologic aging, caused by disease or the results of an unhealthy lifestyle.

This subject is covered more fully in the complete Successful Aging Book

We Age at Different Rates and Earlier Than You Think

External appearance reflects Internal body functions: Signs of aging were already apparent in tests over the 12 years of young adulthood from 26 to 38. The progress of aging happens in our organs just as it does in eyes, joints and hair, but sooner.

Ageing isn't all genetic. Studies of twins found only about 20% of aging is attributed to genes (but some studies now say only 6%), so 80 % to 94% is due to environmental factors, which is what we can change and optimise.

PREMATURE AGING

NORMAL AGING vs. ACCELERATED - PREMATURE AGING

Most "age changes" are, really, premature aging due to abuse, damage or neglect to our bodies.

Premature or Accelerated Aging

While we can see the premature skin aging of sun damage and smoking, we can't see the damage a bad diet and smoking are doing to the insides of our coronary arteries. Even a little amount of sun and smoke, even second-hand smoke, even just one cigarette a day, causes early damage we can and cannot see.

ANTI ACCELERATED-PREMATURE AGING PRINCIPLES

Factors which age people more

1. Smoking
2. Sun
3. Low BMI
4. Low socio-economic class
5. Number of children (men)
6. Marital status
7. Depression (women)
8. High Risk Behaviours / Lifestyle

Prevention
If we *prevent* damage and illness, at all stages and ages, then we optimize health and longevity.
1. Avoidance of High Risk Behaviours - damage
2. Adopting Beneficial Lifestyle
3. Immediately repair even minor damage / illness
4. Identification of Age-Sex Incidence of likely illnesses (All covered in Book 1)

Damage – High Risk Behaviour
'High Risk Behaviours' *are lifestyle habits or actions that increase medical problems.* They are not obviously dangerous escapades, but everyday habits, which account for over 50% of health problems, and include
    Cigarette Smoking
    Eating and Drinking Habits
    Exercise Patterns
    Weight
    Hobbies
    Occupations e.g. sun, exposure, pesticides, pollutants (diesel)
    Sexual Preferences
    Substance abuse
    Medications (sixth greatest cause of premature deaths

Other Factors
    Genes
    Low socio-economic status
    Less affluent neighbourhood / cities
    Pollution

Alternatively, better health optimizes and may delay aging

    Immediate repair to any minor injuries or illnesses
    No major illnesses or complete cure and recovery

Top Risks for deaths, men and women, relevant to all Western Countries:
1. High blood pressure
2. Smoking
3. Overweight / High body mass index
4. High fasting plasma glucose

Drug use is among the fastest growing risk factors for poor health up 53% between 1990 and 2013 and is responsible for the biggest increase in poor health for men. The biggest increase in poor health for women comes from diabetes-related illness increasing by 68% since 1990.

Differences in lifespan in affluent cf disadvantaged areas
A UK has predicted that people living in the longest-living areas in 2012 are expected to live seven or eight years longer than those in disadvantaged. By 2030, the gap is projected to grow to more than eight years even within London and Glasgow suburbs.

Women who lived in the greenest surroundings had a 12% lower overall mortality rate.

MAINTENANCE & PREVENTION

Factors Influencing Health
- Behavioural ~ 50%
- Environment ~ 25%
- Genetic ~ 6 - 25%

Nutrition, Exercise, Environment
1. **Physical**
   - Sun
   - Smoking / substance abuse
   - Overeating / Processed Foods
   - Sedentary lifestyle / unfit
   - Poor nutrition
2. **Mental**
   - Stress
   - Social isolation
   - Lack of mental stimulation / new projects

Types of Intervention
1. **Government legislation & policies**
   There is a line in the sand where people will not tolerate Legislative interference. It is up to you to change your own behaviour
2. **Medical & surgical treatments**
   Have been incredibly successful. Our life expectancy has almost doubled in the last 100 years mostly due to public health measures (clean water etc).
3. **Behavioural Changes – Can People Change?**
   Changing High Risk Behaviour is key to prevention, but Behavioural change results are overwhelmingly disappointing.

CONCLUSIONS

* Most interventions have not worked
* Those that work, have not been implemented
* The present Health Care system is not well designed for successful aging
* It comes down to individual, personal efforts
* People more successful adopting healthy habits if partners do

HEALTH EXPENDITURE

95% of health care spending goes to medical care and research, but lifestyle behaviour and environment are responsible for some 70% of avoidable mortality

PREVENTION PLAN

1. **Maximize Lifestyle**
   - Plan finances – never too early, never too late
   - Think how and where you want to live
   - Assess job opportunities, your suitability and chances
   - Move progressively toward these ambitions. Contentment is often the slow realization of one's aspirations
   - If you want to achieve, mix with achievers

2. **Maximize Health**
   - Minimize Illness
   - Maximize Quality of Life
   - Maximize Longevity
     By identifying and prioritizing
     - The illnesses that most affect us
     - The illnesses that most affect each age group and sex
     - High risk behaviours and bad habits

3. **Empowering individuals to take responsibility for their own health outcomes by**
   - Proven pleasant lifestyle changes and avoiding high risk behaviours
   - Age appropriate investigations to enable early detection of diseases
   - Using results to either effect a cure or minimize the effect of the illness

No substance can extend life (but there are a couple under investigation) but chances of staying healthy and living longer improved by:
- Eating a balanced diet (see Newtrition Super-Mediterranean Diet)
- Exercising regularly
- Getting regular health check-ups (See BOOK 3)
- Stop smoking
- Practise safety habits at home to prevent falls and fractures. Seat belts.
- Keep contact with family, friends. Stay active work, play and community
- Avoid overexposure to the sun and the cold
- Use moderation if you drink. When you drink don't drive
- Keep personal and financial records in order to simplify budgeting and investing. Plan long-term housing and money needs.
- Keep positive attitude toward life. Do things that make you happy.

Repair
* Reduce stress: Opossums Experience on the Mississippi were stressed being attacked by predators. They were wounded, had shorter life spans, stopped breeding but on a predator-free island they flourished.
* Immediate repair to even minor insults
* Back pain core exercises. Muscles waste after just 1 hr of injury / disuse.
* Socio-economic classes – the less education the worse the health
* On-going Preventive Maintenance and checks
* Live Longest Book 3 Age-Specific Illness Identification Killer Lists
* Avoidance of risk behaviour, occupations and hobbies - cars, tractors, ATVs, motor bikes, angle grinders, falls (Book 3)

It is important to understand that being overweight, eating processed and fried foods, and binge drinking are just as much High-Risk Behaviours as smoking, drink-driving and speeding. More than 50%, and probably 70% - 90%, of the factors that adversely affect our health are due to behaviors such as cigarette smoking, poor eating, drinking and exercise patterns. A 'Toxic Environment' no longer means one where there has been a radiation leak or chemical spill. We now live in a 'Toxic Food Environment' where all the wrong kinds of food are available 24 hours-a-day, 7 days a week. Much of this food is high in calories but low in nutritional benefits.

Traffic noise increases the risk of heart attack
Heart attacks increase with road and rail traffic noise, less with aircraft noise.

SLEEP

Results show that one night of partial sleep deprivation activates important biological pathways that promote aging and elevated disease risk.

* People 55-85 did better mental ability tests if they had an afternoon sleep
* Afternoon sleeps (30 min - 2 hrs before 5pm) complemented night sleep
* Siestas reduce heart attacks and sharpen the mind
* Naps may help the immune system to counter sleep restriction damage
* Just make sure it's not due to VAT – Visceral Adipose Tissue (Book 4)

Walking was associated with a decreased likelihood of very short sleep, short sleep and long sleep. Compared with just walking, aerobics/calisthenics, biking, gardening, golf, running, weight lifting, and yoga/Pilates were each associated with decreased likelihood of insufficient sleep, while household/childcare activity was associated with higher.

PHYSICAL

Body image strongly linked to overall life satisfaction

For women, satisfaction with overall appearance was the third strongest predictor, behind financial situation and satisfaction with romantic partner.
For men, appearance satisfaction was the second strongest predictor of life satisfaction, behind only satisfaction with financial situation.
Few men (24%) and women (20%) felt very or extremely satisfied with their weight, and only half felt somewhat to extremely satisfied.

Other key findings included:

- More hours of TV/wk were less satisfied with appearance and weight
- People more satisfied with their appearance and weight had more secure attachment styles, versus fearful and dismissive attachment styles
- People more satisfied with appearance had greater self-esteem, greater life satisfaction, sex life, friends, romantic partners, family, and finances.
- Body Mass Index was strongly related to appearance and dissatisfaction
- Body dissatisfaction and anxious attachment styles can lead to an out of control spiral to fuel each other. People less confident in their appearance become more fearful that their partner will leave, which further fuels their worries about their appearance

Looking Young
Perceived age is a robust biomarker predicting survival for those aged over 70.

Twin Facial Studies
Twins rated younger-looking tended to outlive their older-looking sibling. The bigger the difference in perceived age within a pair, the more likely it was that the older-looking twin died first.

Feeling young at heart may help you live longer
Older people who felt three or more years *younger* than their actual (chronological) age had a lower death rate compared with those who *felt* their age or those who felt more than one year *older* than their actual age.

At age 52 and older, with an average age of 65. Their answers:
- About 70% felt three or more years younger than their actual age
- 25% felt close to their actual age
- 5% felt more than one year older than their actual age

Eight years later those who were still alive:
- 75% of those who felt older than their age
- 82% of those who felt their actual age
- 86% of those who felt younger than their actual age.
- The following have less CardioVascualr (CVS)deaths:
- Younger Looks
* High social status
* Low depression score
* Marriage

Feeling younger may lead to better health habits as in:
1. Exercise: Those who feel old are more likely to abandon physical challenges but those feeling younger psychologically, are more likely to do it.
2. Diet: If we feel young, we may have more of a future-orientation that will lead us to eat with future health in mind and eating better. (Newtrition)

Feeling Older: Disease, Depression and Disuse.
People who feel older are more likely to be hospitalized as they age, regardless of their actual age or other demographic factors and are more likely to be sedentary and to experience faster cognitive decline.

A younger state of mind:
- Try new things, learn new ideas, and develop new skills. Most human abilities follow a "use it or lose it" pattern.
- Appreciate the moment, rather than becoming lost in regrets or imagining future deterioration. Concentrate on the present moment, through mindfulness meditation or informal mindfulness practice.
- Develop a sense of meaning in life. Focus on something larger than yourself: Connect to close friends or help improve lives of others. Commit to a hobby- gardening, the theater, dancing, or reading.

Physical Peak Is Not the End
The Tsimane, of Bolivian Amazonia, despite the harshness of their environment, a combination of physical fitness, limited diet, and immune challenge and reinforcement seem to give them the best heart health observed in any human population with minimal obesity, hypertension, diabetes and peripheral arterial disease and very minimal heart disease. And, while they are a primitive, non-industrialized society, they aren't so different to us. They start aging in their 30s, but physical aging isn't tantamount to decline: Productivity and social status peak long after physical strength and is attributed to adaptation, experience, and maturation for bringing about these late-life benefits

MENTAL

The Paradox of Aging:
The Successful Aging Evaluation (SAGE) study included adults between the ages of 50 and 99 years. Not surprisingly, the oldest adults had worse physical health than their younger counterparts, but they had better mental well-being and scored higher on measures of self-confidence and decision-making skills. Even as physical health deteriorated, mental health quality remained high. Happiness, satisfaction with life went up, levels of depression, stress went down.

The survey concluded that resilience and depression have significant bearing on how individual's self-rate successful aging, with effects that are comparable to that of physical health. In order to flourish, they had to be able to accept and recover from the things they can't change, but also fight for the things they can. The oldest adults had other qualities in common as well, including positivity, a strong work ethic, close bonds with family, religion and the countryside. Most of the older adults in the study were still active, working regularly at home and on their land. This gave them a purpose in life even after they reached old age.

Depressive symptoms increase with age
However, another study showed that depressive symptoms continue to increase throughout old age. It would seem the difference is the mental resilience between the optimists and the pessimists.

> "Two men look out through prison bars,
> One sees mud, one sees stars"

Optimism
Optimists have half the risk of dying from any cause cf pessimists and live 7 years longer, and 1/4 the risk of dying from Cardiovascular Disease - even after adjustments for age, sex, Past Medical History, BMI & other cofounders

Promoting things which evoke a sense of optimism may have a protective role. Depression is the corollary. Positive reinforcement is needed e.g. 'wisdom & creativity' vs. 'senile & dying' which only promotes physical stress and poor mental responses.

Get a Purpose
People with a purpose live longer and are less likely to have large brain infarcts.

Negative Attitude vs. Positive
Older adults with negative attitudes towards aging had slower walking speed and worse cognitive abilities compared to older adults with more positive attitudes.. In the Irish Study TILDA, frail participants with negative attitudes towards aging had worse cognition. However frail participants with positive attitudes towards aging had the same level of cognitive ability as their non-frail peers.

Happiness and unhappiness:
People who think of themselves as unhealthy have a higher mortality.

Recognition, Fulfilment, Contentment
'Success confers a survival advantage'. The corollary of fulfilment is lack of control, frustration and unrequited ambitions i.e. stress which releases damaging kinins. Contentment needn't necessitate achieving former ambitions or recognition but rather *acceptance* of different achievable goals

Life Satisfaction
Greater life satisfaction in adults older than 50 years of age is related to a reduced risk of mortality. If people repeatedly encounter distressing life events that diminish their life satisfaction, such as divorce or unemployment,

then fluctuations in lower levels of satisfaction seem to be particularly harmful for longevity. As participants' life satisfaction increased, the risk of mortality was reduced by 18%. By contrast, greater variability in life satisfaction was associated with a 20% increased risk of mortality. Gardeners live longer

Adaptability
The more one is flexible and adaptable to change the better: The more rigid and resistant to change the worse one ages. As muscles wither without use so does the brain. Furthermore, the narrowing of the brain arteries as we age makes us more inflexible ("set in our ways") which is a negative one-way street and an active pursuit of such challenges should be instituted.

Social Activity Loneliness and Social Isolation
Less social activity is associated with a more rapid rate of motor function decline. The heightened risk of mortality from loneliness is the same as smoking 15 cigarettes a day or being an alcoholic. This surpasses health risks of obesity.

Married Men Don't Have Close Friends: Marriage Cuts Off Friends.
Men being friendless trebles between their early 20s and late middle age. Just over half (51%) when asked how many friends outside their home they would seek to discuss a concern such as money, work or health, said two or fewer, while one in eight said none. Only 7% under 24s said they lacked such close friends, but this rose to 19% over 55s. Married men were more than a third more likely than bachelors to have no close friends outside their home.

The Crisis of Masculinity
There is an alarming rise in suicide among men, especially in middle age.

Social Groups
Membership of social groups after retirement is linked to a longer life, with the impact on health and wellbeing similar to that of regular exercise. Every group membership lost after retirement was associated with around a 10% drop in quality of life score six years later. No such patterns were seen if still employed.

Religious service
Women who attended religious services more than once per week were more than 30% less likely to die. The limitation of the study is that it was of white Christians and included only U.S. nurses of a similar socioeconomic status, who tend to be fairly health conscious. Social support of any kind promotes longer lifespan

Pet Ownership and Health
Compared with people in multi-person households *without* dogs, people living in multi-person households *with* dogs had a risk of death that was 11% lower, and risk of death due to a cardiovascular cause that was 15% lower. For those living alone the risk of death was 33% lower among dog owners, cardiovascular deaths were lower by 36%, and the risk of heart attack was 11% lower.

Retail Therapy
Shopping Malls are free 'clubs' where the isolated and lonely can go and mix and catch up with society trends. It can also be "compensatory consumption". Buying products is a common way to make yourself feel better after a setback. Those who shopped daily were 27% less likely to die. Frequent shopping among the elderly may not be about buying things, but seeking companionship or exercise.

Stress / Bottling It Up / Loneliness
Women who 'self-silenced' during arguments with their husbands are four times more likely to die prematurely than those who speak up for themselves

Marriage
Unmarried men are twice as likely to die as married men. Men with wives who were upset by work were 2.7 times more likely to develop heart disease

Mindfulness (Meditation, Yoga, Nature, Relaxation) beats Exercise
Meditation was prescribed for 20 minutes twice daily. After 5 years of follow-up, a 48% reduction in cardiovascular events was documented. The practice of yoga, consisting of twice-weekly sessions of 1 hour each, reduced the number of episodes of atrial fibrillation by 45%. That said, recent research has found that some people get distressed with meditation. If so, don't do it.

Work
Working Long Hours Linked to Increased Risk for Stroke. Working 55 or more hours per week was associated with a 13% increase in Heart Disease and 33% increase in stroke risk, relative to working 35–40 hours.
Women who worked over 60 hours a week over three decades triple their risk for diabetes, heart trouble and arthritis. The increased risks begin after 40hrs a week.

Driving
Health goes downhill when older adults stop driving doubling the risk of depressive symptoms, along with declines in cognition and physical functioning. Driving cessation was also associated with a 51-percent reduction in the size of social networks of friends and relatives. Former

drivers were also nearly five times as likely as current drivers to be admitted to a nursing home, assisted living community, or retirement home, after adjusting for marital status or co-residence. Merely making alternative transportation available to older adults does not necessarily offset the adverse health effects of driving cessation.

Healthy Survival to 85 for Middle Aged Men

Avoidance of:
- Over-weight
- Hyperglycaemia
- Hypertension
- Smoking
- Excessive alcohol
- Hypertriglyceridemia

Improved survival
- High grip strength
- Marriage

CHAPTER 5.
STAYING SHARP

> **AUTHOR'S NOTE:** Many of these studies are repetitive and duplicating as to their findings. This is both reassuring and 'helpful'(?!).
>
> The ability to learn, solve problems and remember is a key to successful health and aging.

THE AGING BRAIN

Older and Wiser "There are no boy philosophers".
Forgetting names, where you left the keys or appointments only use a small part of the brain. More important is intelligent 'thinking' memory, which works in a different part of the brain and grows with age. 'Stored memory or pattern recognition' allows quicker assessment and solving of problems.

Normal Memory Decline
The decline in memory and brain volume seen in middle age is not due to amyloid plaques and not representative of the first stages of Alzheimer's. It is rather a consequence of normal aging, exacerbated by cerebrovascular disease. Overall, memory worsened from age 30 years through the 90s. Hippocampal volume worsened gradually from age 30 years to the mid-60s and more steeply beyond that age. Amyloid level was low until age 70 years then increased.

Annual Memory Tests for those Over 70.
The recommendation for brain health comes in light of numerous studies, including those in *The Lancet* and *New England Journal of Medicine* that suggest 30% of those older than 70 have memory problems. Approximately 16% of this group has mild cognitive impairment, while 14% has dementia / Alzheimer's.

Some causes of early cognitive disorder can be reversed and treated when caught early. These include depression, hypothyroidism, sleep apnea, problems with sight and hearing, and treatments of multiple health conditions with medications.

SILVER TSUNAMI IOM Report:
Take Action to Promote Brain Health

All first world countries are living longer, however, this aging populace also brings problems: Record numbers of people suffer from dementia, old people are accused of causing road accidents and, in Japan, the police recorded more geriatric offences than juvenile with the cost of looking after the elderly becoming unsustainable for their social security system.

This IOM Cognitive Aging report advises that, outside of the effects of neurologic disease such as Alzheimer's disease, individuals of all ages should take steps to combat the gradual decline in cognitive function that occurs naturally with age.

Four actions "best evidence" for promoting cognitive health all ages;
1. Be physically active.
2. Reduce and manage cardiovascular disease risk factors, including high blood pressure, diabetes, and smoking.
3. Regularly review health conditions and medications that might have a negative effect on cognitive function.
4. Newtrition Super-Mediterranean Foods – No Processed Foods

Other actions, which may promote cognitive health, include:
5. Being socially and intellectually active seeking opportunities to learn.
6. Get adequate sleep and professional treatment for sleep disorders
7. Taking steps to avoid a sudden acute decline in cognitive function (delirium) associated with medications or hospitalizations.
8. Carefully evaluating products advertised to consumers to improve cognitive health, such as medications, nutritional supplements, and cognitive training. No brain supplements work.

The medical literature does not support any vitamin supplement intervention to prevent cognitive decline or the 'neuro-plasticity' commercial programs.

Keeping Sharp vs Age-related Decline
- *Exercise:* People who exercise moderately to vigorously at least once a week are 30% more likely to maintain their cognitive function.
- *Education:* Those who have at least a high school education are nearly three times as likely to stay sharp as those who have less education.
- *Non-smokers:* Are near twice as likely to stay sharp as those who smoke.
- ***Working or volunteering and living with someone:*** Are 24% more likely to maintain cognitive function in late life.

Maintain the Brain
- The brain is the body's most powerful organ
- Muscles lose power lack of use, so can the brain. "Use It or Lose It"
- Brain Resting Energy Expenditure exceeds the heart, kidney or muscles
- Age brings narrowing of arteries and some drop in brain performance
- Never retire. The brain responds to new & different mental challenges
- Retiring at 55 are x2 as likely to die in first 10 years than those work on
- The biggest contributor to function well and properly is our brain

'Cognitive Vitality' Optimised by:
a. Physical fitness / regular exercise
b. Avoidance of high stress
c. Look on the bright side / optimism
d. Rich & varied social life (friends not relatives)
e. Mental stimulation - learn new things
f. Thinking young
g. Newtrition Super-Mediterranean Diet

Mental Challenges
Mentally stimulating activities, like reading, playing games, doing crafts, using the computer and socializing may stave off the development of mild cognitive impairment (MCI).

- Computer use at least once a week was linked to a 42% drop in the risk for memory or thinking issues. About 18% of those who used a computer ended up developing mild cognitive impairment, compared with nearly 31% of seniors who didn't use a computer.
- Reading magazines: 30% drop developing memory and thinking issues.
- Social activities: 23% drop in developing memory impairment.
- Craft tasks e.g. knitting, curtailed the risk of memory problems by 16%
- Game-playing reduced risk by 14%.
- Older adults (>55) who learned multiple new skills at the same time improved their cognitive function to the level of people 30 years younger, two recent small prospective studies showed.

FINGER, a Finnish geriatric study published in *The Lancet*, found those who ate a healthy diet, exercised, trained their memories and managed cardio-vascular risks were less likely to develop cognitive decline and memory problems.

To slow down the progression of not thinking well.
- Mediterranean-type diet -- packed with fruits and vegetables, fish twice a week, olive oil, nuts, legumes and whole grains
- Physical exercise including resistance training, Tai Chi, Dancing,
- Intellectual activity, playing musical instrument less mental decline
- Video games improve reasoning, memory, reaction time and attention

Retirement can be good for health: Leading to positive lifestyle changes
Contrary to the findings that people who retire early die sooner, a major life change like retirement can create a great window of opportunity to make positive lifestyle changes -- it's a chance to get rid of bad routines and engineer new, healthier behaviors.

The data revealed that motivated retirees:
- Increased physical activity by 93 minutes a week
- Decreased sedentary time by 67 minutes per day. The largest reduction was in who lived in urban areas and had higher educational levels
- Increased sleep by 11 minutes per day
- 50% of female smokers stopped smoking

Eating seafood once a week may slow memory loss
Eating seafood or other foods containing omega-3 fatty acids, at least once a week, may protect against age-related memory loss and thinking problems in elderly.

No benefit of omega-3 supplements for cognitive decline
Contrary to popular belief, no benefit of omega-3 supplements for stopping cognitive decline was observed in 4,000 patients followed over a five-year period.

Running barefoot is better than with shoes for memory
Research found a significant increase ~16%, in working memory with barefoot-running but there was no significant increase in working memory when running with shoes. It's possible that the bare feet requires more working memory because of the extra tactile and proprioceptive demands.

Rosemary: The herb enhances memory. **Lavender** makes people soporific.

STRESS and BURNOUT
Symptoms and Signs
- Feeling physically and emotionally exhausted, drained, and depleted
- Loss of enjoyment. Pessimism.
- Forgetfulness/impaired concentration and attention.
- Increasing cynicism and detachment
- Progressive isolation
- Feelings of ineffectiveness, lack of accomplishment and not coping
- Physical symptoms - palpitations, difficulty breathing, headaches
- Increased illness, especially colds due to weakened immune system
- Loss of appetite
- Increased irritability with outbursts of anger
- "I need a holiday"
- Suicide hints
- Seek help immediately if you are experiencing any of the following.
- Don't put it off.

CHAPTER 6.
DEMENTIA and ALZHEIMER DISEASE

Dementia vs. Alzheimer's (AD)
Again this may be somewhat repetitive from the last chapter as there is overlap.

Dementia and Alzheimer's disease are not the same.

Dementia
According to the American National Institute on Aging (NIA), Dementia is *an umbrella term* for a set of symptoms. It is a syndrome (a group of symptoms), not a disease that affects mental cognitive tasks such as memory and reasoning. It is a chronic neuro-degenerative disorder characterized clinically by deterioration of daily living, behavioral functioning, and global cognitive ability.

It can occur due to a variety of conditions, the most common of which is Alzheimer's disease. People can have more than one type of dementia. This is known as mixed dementia which can only be confirmed in an autopsy.

The spectrum ranges from mild cognitive impairment to the neurodegenerative diseases of Alzheimer's, cerebrovascular disease, Parkinson's disease and Lou Gehrig's (Motor Neuron) disease. Furthermore, many types of memory may decline with aging, but not semantic memory or general knowledge whereas episodic memory consists of personal facts and experience e.g. knowing that football is a sport is an example of semantic memory but recalling what happened during the last football game that you attended is an episodic memory.

Causes of dementia
It occurs when certain brain cells are damaged. Many conditions can cause dementia; each causes damage to a different set of brain cells.
- **Alzheimer's** accounts for 62% of cases
- **Vascular Dementia** caused by restricted blood supply = 17%
- **Other causes of dementia include:**
  Infections, HIV   Vitamin deficiencies
  Vascular diseases   Neurological Diseases
  Stroke   Diet and inactivity
  Depression   Anticholinergics
  Chronic drug use

Symptoms of dementia

It's easy to overlook the early symptoms of dementia, which can be mild. It often begins with simple episodes of forgetfulness, keeping track of time and tend to lose their way in familiar settings. Forgetfulness and confusion grow. It is harder to recall names and faces. Personal care becomes a problem.

Obvious signs of dementia include
- repetitious questioning
- inadequate hygiene
- poor decision-making

In the most advanced stage
- people with dementia become unable to care for themselves
- they struggle even more with keeping track of time and remembering people and places they are familiar with
- behaviour changes continue and can turn into depression and aggression

Alzheimer Disease (AD)

Alzheimer disease is a very specific form of dementia that specifically affects parts of the brain that control thought, memory and language. It causes as many as 50 to 70% of all dementia cases. It is a progressive disease that slowly causes impairment in memory and cognitive function. The exact cause is unknown.

Alzheimer's vs. Dementia symptoms

The symptoms of Alzheimer's and Dementia can overlap, but there can be some differences.

Both conditions can cause:
- A decline in the ability to think
- Memory impairment
- Communication impairment

The symptoms of Alzheimer's include:
- Difficulty remembering recent events or conversations
- Apathy
- Depression
- Impaired judgment
- Disorientation
- Confusion
- Behavioural changes
- Difficulty speaking, swallowing, or walking in advanced stages

Diagnosis: Blood Test
A blood test that may be up to 94% accurate in finding people with early Alzheimer's brain changes has been developed.

The Effects of Alzheimer's on the Brain
Damage to the brain begins years before symptoms appear.

It's impossible to diagnose Alzheimer's with complete accuracy while a person is alive and can only be confirmed by an autopsy. However, specialists are able to make the correct diagnosis up to 90% of the time.

The underlying pathology of Alzheimer's makes any cure most unlikely. It would seem the best we can do is get in early with preventive measures, such as they are. and you may wish to try the following:
- Exercise training combined with behavioural management improves physical health and depression in Alzheimer's
- Diversity of exercise rather than intensity seems more protective
- Some Authorities claims that the combination of a good diet and exercise postpone deterioration by 40%.

People with gout, but not those with simple osteoarthritis, are 24-29% less likely to develop AD. Is uric acid, which causes gout, protective?

Treatment / Prevention
Obviously, no one knows the cause(s) and there is no definitive treatment. However, our brains, like our muscles, have a natural shrinkage and like our muscles respond to usage. Exercise increases the blood flow to the brain. Brisk walking for an hour twice a week increased cognition while playing a hand-eye sport, such as table tennis, improved critical thinking. Dancing is one of the best overall exercises working all muscle groups. Learning a new skill, such as a new language or painting, challenges and improves the brain.

> *Early education and life experience protect*
> Elaborate writing style x3 less likely to develop Alzheimer's
> The greater the Grammatical Complexity the less Alzheimer's
> Never too late to keep exercising mind - promotes and protects
> *Lifestyle*
> Less stress
> Diet: Less meat more fruit and veg- Newtrition Diet
> No processed foods: Perhaps it is a bit of a hobby-horse of mine but obesity and dementia do seem to shadow the increase in processed foods. I think "we can't process processed foods" and there are now 87,000 chemical supplements many of which are in junk food. Maybe these get through our blood-brain barrier to deposit.
> *Angiotensin receptor II blockers (ARBs)*
> ARBs for hypertension improved long-term memory-related outcomes

and a smaller volume of white-matter hyperintensities and are probably associated with greater memory preservation and less white-matter volume than other antihypertensive medications.

Social contact,
in middle age and late life, appears to lower the risk of dementia. A person who saw family and friends almost every day had a 12 per cent lower risk of developing conditions such as Alzheimer's disease.

Exercise / Physical Activity
Exercise and cardio-vascular health provide protection against cognitive decline. 8,300 steps were enough. More was better.

Dental Hygiene
Research has found that people with periodontal disease are at higher risk for AD. Some studies have shown that gum disease precedes AD, which means bacterial infection precedes the onset of AD rather than AD causing neglect of dental hygiene. See your dentist every six months for cleaning.

Choline
A new study (published August 2019) has shown that dietary intake of phosphatidylcholine is associated with a reduced risk of dementia. Phosphatidylcholine was also linked to enhanced cognitive performance. The main dietary sources of phosphatidylcholine were eggs and meat.

Low and High Haemaglobin
Individuals with anemia were 41% more likely to develop Alzheimer's disease (AD) and 34% more likely to develop any dementia type and, in addition, those with high hemoglobin were also at greater risk of developing dementia.

Good cardiovascular (CV) health
Good cardiovascular (CV) health in middle age face lower risk for dementia in older age. During a median follow-up of 25 years, 4% of participants developed dementia. After multivariable adjustment, each additional optimal metric (e.g., being a nonsmoker) was associated with a significant, 12% decrease in dementia risk.

Ultra-processed foods
It is widely recognised that type 2 diabetes (T2D) represents a major disease burden but it is only recently that its role in neurodegeneration has attracted more attention. This research has shown that T2D is associated with impaired cerebral health, cognitive decline and dementia. Processed foods are thought to contribute to development of T2D. Basic advice is to avoid food and drinks listing multiple complex chemicals on their labels.

Okinawa
50% less dementia than the West
80% reduced CVD
Uschi ghushi - food is medicine
Vegetables - sweet potatoes - purple - 0.5 kg a day
Eat moderately (leave food on the plate and never feel full)

Benefit of respect: Respect for elderly written into Japanese law
Food: See Newtrition Super-Mediterranean Diet
Purple vegetables good - purple Sweet Potato = ancocyanins seem to boost blood flow. Blueberries, blackcurrants, egg-plant, purple cabbage
Exercise
Dancing
General Health
Keeping healthy in middle age is important for brain aging and reducing risk of dementia in old age.

Midlife activity and dementia

- After 44 years middle aged Swedish women who were most active at the time they entered the study were the least likely to suffer dementia in old age. Cognitive activity in midlife reduced the risk of Alzheimer's disease, while physical activity reduced the risk of mixed and vascular dementia.
- Exercise and weight loss improves glucose regulation, better memory
- Exercise and fish rich diet maintain memory / slowed brain aging: 1 fish meal a week = 10% pa slower. 2 fish meals = 13 % slower decline.
- Aged over 90 most people's memory remains good
- Well educated people aged 75 + often outperformed those aged 50 + as to mental tasks
- But being smart does not necessarily confer contentment or happiness
- Cognitive vitality, contentment are necessary for successful aging – optimum lifespan
- Early adult psychological disorders are associated with increased mortality
- 30% soccer players had memory problems cf 10% swimmers. Soccer players also had smaller brains, more Parkinson's disease and other neurological problems (the long term sequalae of even minor head injuries is now being recognised)
- A higher level of daily physical activity was tied to slower amyloid-beta (Aβ)-related cognitive decline (Alzheimer's). Even modest levels of physical activity had robust protective effects, but they were most prominent in people who took about 8,900 steps a day.
- Living a healthy lifestyle was associated with a reduced dementia risk regardless of genetic risk. Individuals at high genetic risk who followed an unhealthy lifestyle were almost three times more likely to develop dementia within 8 years than those with a low genetic risk and a favourable lifestyle.

Healthy Heart, Healthy Brain
Having more ideal cardiovascular health factors was associated with better brain processing speed at the study's start and less cognitive decline.

Drugs for Dementia and Circulation
No type of medicine seems to work better than another.
Eating a large amount of fatty foods and living in a polluted area may increase dementia risk. Some dementia, such as a drug interactions or vitamin deficiency, are reversible or temporary. Atrial Fibrillation, an increasingly common heart arrythmia in those over 60 is linked to an increased risk of developing Dementia. Get an ECG/EKG.
In the first trial intranasal insulin may be effective in slowing progression of mild cognitive impairment (MCI) or Alzheimer's disease (AD) by 1 to 2 years but it depends on the delivery device and more research is needed. Insulin can penetrate the blood-brain barrier.

Falling Incidence
Despite the perception that Dementia and Alzheimer's is increasing, it has fallen by 22% in those over 65 from 8.3% to 6.5%. While the proportion has fallen the number of cases has increased because there are more, older people. The impact of dementia is still huge- around 7% of people over 65 and 40% of those over 80.

The falling numbers are largely thought to be driven by improved education and living conditions, better prevention and treatment of vascular and chronic conditions and people exercising more, giving up smoking, and switching to more nutritious diets, suggesting that up to 30% might be preventable.

Influenza vaccinations may improve dementia and other Health Outcome
Patients who had the flu vaccine had a 35% lower risk of developing dementia vs. those who never received the vaccine. In addition, *the dementia risk was 55% lower in those who had received at least three doses over the previous years.*

Specific brain training reduces dementia risk across 10 years
While many systems have long promised that their brain-training products can sharpen aging minds, only one or two types of computerized brain training so far has been shown to improve people's mental quickness and significantly reduce the risk of dementia.

Brain Stimulation
Learning a new skill - best - challenge the brain

A second language increases different parts of the Brain

Drawing - a new subject each time

Early education and life experience seem to donate protection. Those demonstrating elaborate writing style are three times less likely to develop Alzheimer's; the greater their grammatical complexity the less Alzheimer's. And it's never too late to keep exercising the mind, which promotes and protects it.

Stress is also destructive and must be minimized.

Boosting Levels of Antioxidant Glutathione May Help Resist Age-Related Decline. Glutathione helps resist the toxic stresses of everyday life -- but its levels decline with age and this sets the stage for a wide range of age-related health problems. The compound -- N-acetyl-cysteine, or NAC -- is known to boost the metabolic function of glutathione and increase its rate of synthesis.

Less Teeth More Dementia
Individuals with less than 20 teeth were at a 20% higher risk for developing cognitive decline and dementia than those with greater than or equal to 20 teeth.

There may be relationships between oral inflammation, gum disease, systemic inflammatory burden, and cognitive status.

Low Vitamin D Linked to Cognitive Decline
Low vitamin D levels are very common in older adults, especially African Americans and Hispanics, and are associated with accelerated decline in episodic memory and executive function, the two cognitive domains strongly associated with Alzheimer's disease (AD) dementia. The magnitude of the effect of Vitamin D insufficiency on cognition was substantial. It is suggested measuring vitamin D status in older patients and supplements if warranted. Do not take otherwise.

Pollution

Particles known as PM2.5 are minute, invisible, sooty bits of combustion that are key culprits in the air pollution health crisis as they are small enough to make it deep into the lungs and from there into the bloodstream. Studies show such pollution is linked in adults to cancers, lung disease, hypertension, heart attacks and strokes.

They are produced by diesel and petrol fumes, log burners and even conventional ovens.

The cocktail of chemicals in PM2.5 particles, in combination with other pollutants like nitrogen and sulphur dioxides, impacts brain function with increased systemic inflammation, which damages the blood vessels supplying the brain. It is suggested that volatile chemicals attack the hormone-producing endocrine system, disrupting normal physical development.

A large 2019 study concluded: "Early life exposure to PM2.5 was associated with a reduction in fundamental cognitive abilities, including working memory and attention.

In 2018, a London study found those in the most polluted areas were 40 per cent more likely to be diagnosed with dementia.

In 2017, a huge analysis of more than 2 million people found another correlation between pollution and dementia in London, stating that 7 per cent of dementia cases could be attributed to "elevated pollution exposure".

Pollution is not just confined to the Cities. All volatile compounds, like pesticides found in rural areas, can be included and there may be a geographical pattern specific to dementia, and potentially Alzheimer's. Lifestyle and genes all play their part but where you live may also be a factor for our long-term brain health.

Basic Advice
- Avoid main roads and busy streets.
- Face masks don't work as they don't keep out the smallest particulate matter, which is most damaging.
- Walk on the opposite side from the kerb as pollution levels can be more than a third higher on the kerb side of the pavement. If you are waiting to cross at a busy junction, Greenpeace suggests pressing the cross button then taking several steps back.
- Exposure to pollution may be worse inside cars than outside; walking or cycling is healthier than driving.
- If you must drive, close windows and air vents. Drivers and passengers in the middle of the road suffer most and keeping air vents closed in busy traffic could help reduce exposure.
- Open windows away from street front or potential prevailing polluted winds.

CHAPTER 7.

POLLUTANTS AND ENDOCRINE DISRUPTING CHEMICALS (EDC)

The Madrid Statement of 2015.
200 scientists from various disciplines signed a statement expressing concerns as to all fluro-chemicals (PFASs). These are used in the manufacture of pesticides, plastics and petrol. Even low doses can cause cancer, thyroid problems and nervous system disorders. The scientists recommended avoiding products that are stain-resistant, waterproof or non-stick. While heavy metals and pesticide dangers are well known there is concern that some of these EDCs are not safe.

Microwaving food in plastic: Dangerous or not?
The FDA long ago recognized the potential for small amounts of plasticizers to migrate into food. So, it closely regulates plastic containers and materials that come into contact with food. When Good Housekeeping microwaved food in 31 plastic containers, lids, and wraps, it found that almost none of the food contained plastic additives.

Is Styrofoam microwave safe? Contrary to popular belief, some Styrofoam and other polystyrene containers can safely be used in the microwave. Just follow the same rule you follow for other plastic containers: Check the label.

Here are some things to keep in mind when using the microwave:
- If you're concerned about plastic wraps or containers in the microwave, transfer food to glass or ceramic containers labeled for use in microwave ovens.
- Don't let plastic wrap touch food during microwaving because it may melt. Wax paper, kitchen parchment paper, white paper towels, or a domed container that fits over a plate or bowl are better alternatives.
- Most takeout containers, water bottles, and plastic tubs or jars made to hold margarine, yogurt, whipped topping, and foods such as cream cheese, mayonnaise, and mustard are not microwave-safe.
- Microwavable takeout dinner trays are formulated for one-time use only and will say so on the package.
- Old, scratched, or cracked containers, or those that have been microwaved many times, may leach out more plasticizers.
- Don't microwave plastic storage bags or plastic bags from the grocery store. Before microwaving food, be sure to vent the container: leave the lid ajar or lift cover edge.

CHAPTER 8.
MEDICATIONS

Most prescribed medications are necessary but four major problems:
1. Taking the wrong dosage or mixing too many
2. Adding in a new one and not trying to reduce the number
3. Not taking them
4. Potential dangerous side-effects

An annual review of all medications, and any supplements, should be done.

Minimally Disruptive Medicine (MDM)
It is universally acknowledged that many older people take too many drugs, and that many are being harmed by taking the wrong drugs or the wrong combination of drugs. The American Geriatrics Society publishes the *'Beers Criteria for Potentially Inappropriate Medication Use in Older Adults'* and, from my perusal it looks excellent – even if you are not old but have been prescribed one of the listed drugs. No doctor can keep track of all the medications and this provides a double check. www.americangeriatrics.org.

Americans >65yrs have 8% chance being prescribed inappropriate drugs.
A UK study found that between 1995 and 2010 the proportion of adults dispensed five or more and 10 or more drugs doubled to 20.8% and tripled to 5.8%, respectively. The proportion with potentially serious drug-drug interactions more than doubled to 13%.
More elderly using dangerous drug combinations
One in six older adults now regularly use potentially deadly combinations of prescription and over-the-counter medications and dietary supplements.

Published and unpublished data of some new drugs
50% of all new drugs have important side effects discovered only after approval and marketing. Unfortunately, the results of trials in which a new drug performs better than existing drugs are more likely to be published than those in which the new drug performs badly or has unwanted side effects (publication bias). Moreover, trial outcomes that support the use of a new treatment are more likely to be published than those that do not support its use (outcome reporting bias). The Drug Companies are becoming increasingly competitive and profit motivated such that essential information has been withheld or suppressed.

Under-prescribing Adds to Mortality, Hospitalization Among Oldest Old
Inappropriate under-prescribing of medications is associated with increased mortality and hospitalization rates among community-dwelling adults aged 80 years and older. Patients with five or more medications (a standard cut-off used for polypharmacy) can have a well-tailored and balanced medication therapy with an acceptable risk for adverse events.

Yet, in contrast, patients with just a few medications could be at risk missing essential and beneficial medications. Two-thirds of the population had underuse, 56.1% had misuse, and only 17.1% had neither underuse nor misuse. Four in 10 participants (40.2%) had a combination of underuse with misuse.

Drugs don't work in patients who don't take them
There is an out-of-control epidemic in the US that costs more and affects more people than any disease Americans currently worry about. It's called non-adherence to prescribed medications, and it is — potentially, at least — 100% preventable by the very individuals it afflicts.

The numbers are staggering. "Studies have consistently shown that 20% to 30% of medication prescriptions are never filled, and that approximately 50% of medications for chronic disease are not taken as prescribed." This lack of adherence is estimated to cause approximately 125,000 deaths and at least 10% of hospitalizations, and to cost the American health care system between $100 billion and $289 billion a year.

MEDICATIONS TO WATCH – Refer to the Complete Book 3.

Antidepressants
    The tricyclic antidepressants, such as doxepin or amitriptyline, even when used at low doses for migraine prevention or neuropathic pain
Antibiotics
Anticholinergics
    Memory and reasoning tests were worse in those taking them.
    May increase dementia rate by 50%. Scans showed less cortical volume These drugs implicated are commonly used, estimated to be taken by about 20% of the older adult population for many conditions. They include popular antihistamines sold over the counter as sleep aids, such as diphenhydramine, or for allergy relief, such as chlorpheniramine; oxybutynin and tolterodine for overactive bladder.
Anti-Hypertensives
Aspirin

PPI (Protein Pump Inhibitors for Heartburn)
Statins
Anxiolytics and Sleeping Tablets
NSAIDS

UNPROVEN 'REJUVENATORS': 'DISEASE MONGERING'

Please consult the complete book for details.

Disease mongering is inventing new wider definitions of conditions in conjunction with aggressive marketing to increase sales of some drugs and therapies, usually for contrived entities they were not designed to initially treat. e.g. The mass marketing of testosterone by innuendo and advertising which encouraged using testosterone for anti-aging rather than actual proven deficiency.

Disease Mongering Inventions
- *DHEA (Dehydropiandrosterone)*
- *Growth Hormone (hGH)*
- *Growth Hormone Secretagogues (e.g. Capromorelin)*
- *Melatonin*
- *Testosterone*
- *HRT*
- *Vitamins, Supplements and Antioxidants*

Longevity expert Thomas Perls, MD, MPH, a professor of medicine at the Boston University School of Medicine, characterizes the prescribing of human growth hormone (HGH) for anti-aging as "quackery and hucksterism" and that hormone replacement therapy and the drugs used to treat their side effects end up being hormonal toxic soups that can cause great medical and financial harm that far outweighs any long-term benefit.

Some Evidence
- *Western Medicines:*
    Metformin, Selegiline, ACE inhibitors

Metformin is a diabetes medication to manage insulin resistance. Patients who have taken the drug have less cancer, less heart disease, and less frailty than the average population. There are proposed trials but funding is proving a problem. It has been found, however that can blunt certain physical changes from exercise that normally help people to age well.

The results raise questions about the relationship of pills and physical activity in healthy aging and also whether we know enough about how drugs and exercise interact.

Proceed with caution.

- ***Calorie Restriction***

Conclusions

Best advice is to 'wait and see'

Long term side effects often reveal themselves far removed from the original purpose e.g. Thalidomide, Vioxx

All supplements are snake-oil quackery - don't do yourself harm, or waste money

Eat fresher, better and exercise more.

Healthy food, incidentally, is not labelled 'healthy'.

CHAPTER 9.
SEX

Both desire and drive (libido) and performance reduce with age, but it can still be satisfying, and many older people continue to enjoy their sexuality into their 80s and beyond. A healthy sex life not only is fulfilling, but also is good for other aspects of life, including physical health and self-esteem.

Many older couples report greater satisfaction with their sex life because they have fewer distractions, more time and privacy, and no worries about pregnancy. Sex may not have the same intensity as when you were younger can continue to be a rewarding part of your life.

Peoples' libidos go from neutral, where they hardly have any sex urge to rampant sexual "addiction" for want of a better term, but the male is far more active in this regard. There is no medical "recommendation" as to how much and how often sex at any age is to be had.

The Elephant in the Room
The problem not addressed and not voiced is that when women menopause they lose their desire (libido) while men continue to want sex.

WHAT TO DO

Both
Discuss: Come to a Mutual Agreement
Unless both parties needs and desires are frankly discussed then the potential is to only get worse. Male patients have expressed to me their complete bewilderment and frustration at their former sexy partner now being frigid. The scenario where the woman is subjected to demands she simply does not feel like is untenable: The scenario where the man is denied and cut out is also untenable.

The hope and the best way forward is an English Report which identifies that older (menopaused) women can and do enjoy sex or, at least, "were least likely to express dissatisfaction" even if they "had less of it or minded about it less".

A frank discussion can avoid the woman feeling harassed and the man more understanding and less demanding.

Expand your horizons: **Foreplay,** fondling, touching, stroking, kissing and other intimate contact are probably more needed now than when you were young. It also alerts your partner and helps set the mood. As you age, it's normal for you and your partner to have different sexual abilities and needs. Be open to finding new ways to enjoy sex.

Alter Set Routines: There is nothing less stimulating or more stultifying that a set routine for sex. Not too many young people so indulged! Be impulsive. Change. Change the time of day. Change positions or explore other ways of connecting romantically and sexually. The bedroom isn't the only place.

Romance: Part and parcel of the above is that set routines are like throwing cold water whereas romance is like lighting the fire. Think of what used to "turn you on" when you were courting: You haven't changed that much! Re-activate!

While initially this may be difficult in time a new desire and libido will re-establish - especially if the couple have a good relationship otherwise.

Women
In this present movement for female equality, with which I agree, I do think, however, the French observation "vive la difference" has been suppressed. Men and women *are* different - obviously - and one big difference, not usually emphasized, is that men want sex more than women. That said, living on a farm as we do, few of the cows and bitches are definitely more "vigorous" than others.

This is animal-tribal survival. Humans are the only animal who can mate and breed in any season. All other females have to "come into season" but where the human female differs from the male is that when she gets pregnant or menopauses, her libido drops whereas the males' keeps going.

What this means is that your libido as a young person is as part of your personality as any other trait and as you age so it will too. This may require some re-adjustment between couples with menopause.

Menopause brings a sudden stop to the previous cycle of hormones and a reduction in desire for sex. Postmenopausal women, have lower levels of the hormone estrogen, which in turn decreases vaginal lubrication and elasticity. In many cases, dryness can be relieved by something as simple as using a water-based lubricant like KY Jelly. Doctors offer other remedies for difficult cases.
Warning: Oestrogen creams used to soften the vaginal mucosa and as a lubricant can transfer to the man with feminising effects.

Men

For men a different problem arises or, to be more accurate, doesn't rise as they have progressive loss of erections. Testosterone levels decline slowly but not suddenly cut off like womens' hormones with menopause. Changes in sexual function are common such as:

- Impotence or have more difficulty achieving and sustaining erections as their blood circulation slows and testosterone levels decrease. Impotence is also more prevalent in men who have a history of heart disease, hypertension, or diabetes.
- A need for more stimulation to achieve and maintain erection and orgasm
- Shorter orgasms
- Less forceful ejaculation and less semen ejaculated
- Longer time needed to achieve another erection after ejaculation

Health Issues

Illnesses can have a big effect on sex life and sexual performance. You and your partner will now have to experiment with ways to adapt to your limitations. It is no time to be coy - "it takes two to tango" and it's a problem for both of you...to solve. **Above all talk with your partner e**ven if it is difficult and embarrassing. Only by sharing your needs, desires and concerns can help you both enjoy sex and intimacy more.If you're worried about sex after a heart attack, talk with your doctor. With arthritis, try different positions or using heat to alleviate joint pain.

Medications

Blood pressure tablets, antihistamines, antidepressants and acid-blocking drugs (PPIs), can all affect sexual function.

Impotence

Sildenafil citrate (Viagra), vardenafil (Levitra), and tadalafil (Cialis) have offered a significant breakthrough. They don't work for all men and not as well as rumor or manufacturers would have you think. Not all men, especially those with angina, can have them. Check with your doctor.

Depression

Paradoxically Depression can increase the desire for and interest in sex. On the other hand, it can manifest a profound disinterest. On both counts it's time for help but Anti-depressants are anti-sex and, in any event, I am not a fan of them.

Anxiety

Aging brings on inevitable unavoidable changes with which we have to come to terms. But, in addition, there are those which strike us "out of left field"- from the death of your partner to financial problems. As to finances, it may well be a time to downsize and grow closer. Easier said than done but if you have each other you seriously don't need all that money and sex is, after all, free.

CHAPTER 10.
PREPARING FOR OLD AGE: Begin in your 40s.

Plan Ahead. While it may be an exaggeration to begin in your 40s, give some thought to where and how you want to live before you invest. Moving to the country can entail unforeseen problems which initially can be coped with, but later present a problem such as longer commuting with more downtime, more expense and increased traffic accidents.

While a swimming pool and a tennis court are good in your old age, who maintains them? But the big issue are high rise houses with stairs. I am a fan of stairs as they impose one of the most beneficial exercises, but they are also a source of increasing injuries as we age. Have an exit strategy before you can't cope, break a hip and need to be closer to a hospital.

Eventually you won't be able to do what you currently do such as driving, shopping, cleaning, managing finances or medications. Have lists of trusted trades and repairmen.

Home modifications. Convenient public transport increasingly important. Stairs, baths may need rails or a one-story place.

Prevent falls. Being aware of the danger is of greatest importance. Never stand on chairs or ladders to hang curtains or such. Beware of tiled slippery floors. Get checked for osteoporosis. Always use hand-rails.

Emergencies. Get someone to check on you regularly? Carry a mobile / cellphone. Practice using it. Have emergency numbers coded into speed dial.

Advance care directives. Make a living will, durable power of attorney.

Adequate Finances: Poverty levels depend on several factors, including the adequacy of the pension systems and the age and sex structure of the elderly population, since elderly women and very old people are more likely to live in poverty. Adequate financial resources are important. Poverty is defined as 60% of the respective country's median income.

Financial Scams: Cognitive aging has significant effects and widespread consequences on society, including financial losses, with older adults losing an estimated $2.9 billion annually, directly and indirectly, to financial fraud.

Medical History / Records Legal Issues: Ensure your Power of Attorney, will, health directives as to your wishes (e.g. DNR- Do Not Resuscitate) are easily located and known to others. Originals will be needed. Carry a medical history / medication list on you plus the location.

Be Flexible - in Body and Mind: Back pain is one of the most prevalent of human conditions with many causes. It gets worse as we get older no matter the cause. But it means we have progressive difficulty accessing our toes. Cutting our toenails or putting on socks and stockings becomes very difficult as is putting on underpants, trousers and slacks.

Yoga itself may be the way to go. Tai Chi is another that promotes flexibility.

But do flexibility exercises daily or you will "freeze-up".

Elsewhere I have pointed out how the narrowing of our cerebral arteries leads to progressively more rigid behavior...things such as the tooth brush and such *"must"* always be in the same place or these old people cannot cope with any such changes. We cannot stop this arteriosclerosis at this stage but forewarned is forearmed and if we notice our progressive mental inflexibility we may be able to combat it and relax more. Beware of fixed ideas and rigid behaviors.

Posture: We all know elderly people become stooped. Our "perfect posture" is when we stand against a wall and push our calves, bottom, shoulders and back of head into the wall and suck in our stomachs.

Our necks progressively tilt forward with age (just have a look around) and this pushes our neck vertebrae into our esophagus such that we are more prone to have food or drink "go down the wrong way" and we choke. The best posture is "chin-in and imagine someone pulling you scalp hair up to the ceiling". Walk tall.

Hospitals: 1 in 3 Worse off when discharged. Keep Walking! Keep Mobile!
Patients admitted to hospital expect to leave in a better state, but in practice this isn't always the case: One in three patients aged 70 and older were discharged from the hospital with functional decline and around one in two report a decline in functioning a month after their discharge.

One of the main factors leading to functional decline was reduced mobility while in the hospital. Patients often mistakenly think that if they're sick, they ought to be in bed, and around half of the patients didn't leave their rooms during their entire hospital stay.

On average, study participants reported consuming only 60% of the recommended daily calories during their hospitalization. The reasons for reduced nutrition included the unfamiliar taste of the food, a lack of appetite, and periods of fasting needed before various tests.

There is an increased risk of death of 10% for admissions on a Saturday and 15% for admissions on a Sunday compared with patients admitted on a Wednesday.

Nursing Home: Take Your Own Fruit and Veg!
People who became residents of nursing homes and fed the unrelenting same diet soon had a less diverse gut microbiome and were more likely to be frail and suffer from illnesses and to die within a year. It is thought the main culprit appears to be the lack of fresh fruit and vegetables.

WARNING DANGER AHEAD:

Lifespans are exceeding economic plans.

While we have desperately embraced the pursuit of *'staying young and having fun'* we have neglected most other aspects of *successful aging* from both economic and social aspects. People are now putting aside fewer savings for old age than they have in any decade since the Great Depression. More than half the old live without a spouse and we have fewer children than ever before. Yet we give virtually no thought how we will live out our later years alone.

In the USA when the cost for a decent retirement community was $30,000 pa, the annual income for those over 80 was only $15,000. More than half the elderly who live in long-term care facilities go through their entire savings and have to go on welfare and ultimately spend a year or more in a nursing home at twice the cost. People still look forward to retiring at 65 years or even younger. This is a sad goal, and many learn to rue the day as their lives descend into an unstimulating existence. But while it may have been economically feasible when those over 65 comprised a minute fraction of society it is simply not so when they will soon make up more than 20% of society.

Multifactorial
The most recent enthusiasm is in analyzing the gut microbiome as above where a reduced biome due to poor nutrition is associated with deterioration and even death. Twin studies provide a good basis for much of this evidence. However, other studies also blame the reduced mobility, medications especially sleeping tablets as well as more obvious interferences such as in-dwelling catheters.

Frailty, which is what they all measure, is a significant sign as to a person's deterioration and a harbinger of mortality and while it would seem poor nutrition plays its part, in some cases one is left to wonder which came first the frailty or the poor nutrition and reduced mobility / exercise.

CHAPTER 11.
INTIMATIONS of MORTALITY: MOMENTO MORI

Predicting Death
Data from nearly half a million men, ages 40 to 52, who said they had a slow walk speed, revealed that they had a 3.7 times higher risk for overall mortality when compared with men in the same age range who reported brisker speeds. My interpretation of this data is that it is not the faster walking per se but the fact that the person is fitter and healthier that ensures they walk faster. So, if you are a slow walker go and get fit!

A previous cancer diagnosis was the strongest predictor of all-cause mortality in women, Lung cancer was the leading cause of death in men while breast cancer was the leading cause of death in women out of 498,103 participants, ages 37 to 73, who were included in the analysis.

The study also reaffirmed the evidence that increases in physical activity, smoking cessation, and having a healthy diet can increase longevity.

A Good Death
Everyone agreed that it is important to make preferences for the dying process known, such as where you want to die, and everyone wants it be pain-free, but after that, determining what is a good death was less uniform. Eleven "core themes" of a good death have been identified: Preferences for a specific dying process:
1. Dying during sleep
2. Having advanced directives in place
3. Pain-free status
4. Religiosity/spirituality
5. Emotional well-being
6. Life completion
7. Treatment preferences
8. Dignity
9. Family
10. Quality of life
11. Relationship with Health Care Provider
12. "Other."

The top three core themes were
1. Preferences for dying process (94% of the studies/reports)
2. Pain-free status (81%)
3. Emotional well-being (64%).

BOOK 3

WHAT'S GOING TO KILL YOU THIS YEAR?

(And how to avoid them)

Live Longer Healthier

Chronic conditions, not infectious diseases, are top 5 causes of early death.

Most of these can be prevented, avoided, treated and minimized

---

Only 8% of us get correct Preventive advice

Medical care prevents only 10% of premature deaths

Healthy behaviours and lifestyle can improve this to 65%

The Live Longest Preventive Advice may improve this to 90%

It uniquely identifies the risks for your age & how to avoid them

SECTION A

CHAPTER 1.
WHAT'S MISSING (TO ALLOW US LIVE LONGER)?

Everyone knows how to live longer...or do they?

The good advice is not to smoke, eat well, minimise alcohol, maintain optimum weight, control blood pressure and cholesterol and exercise.

This "good advice" is indeed good, but it lacks the finer details that those who live longer actually practice. Some of these good practices are enforced by the community in which they live, known as "The Blue Zones" (see Chapter 14), but, for most of us, modern urban lifestyles mitigate against these enforced practices.

However, there has been one glaring omission: ***The big glaring omission*** has been identifying what risks and illnesses are *age-specific*. What kills or disables us in our 20's are not the same as those in our 40's and so on for each decade.

These are the Missing Keys or, to emphasise their importance, *<u>just what are the risks or illnesses that are the most likely to kill or disable you this year.</u>*

While most of this information, has been available in isolated specialities and research, they haven't been sourced and then collated into one 'package' to allow you to maximise and employ these age-specific alerts...until now.

In addition:
- How come diabetes 2 is an epidemic?
- How come obesity is an epidemic?
- How come heart disease is preventable but has been, and still is, our greatest killer?
- How come then, that most people over the age of 60 have three chronic diseases?
- How come most of us will be a premature shambling wreck, taking 10 medications a day and committed to a nursing home before we die prematurely?

<u>These are the actual official statistics,</u> and this is where you are headed.

Unless you take the correct steps to prevent them. Read on.

CHAPTER 2.
PREMATURE DEATHS OVERVIEW

Death after the age of 80 years is the ambition and is not "Premature".

Tobacco use then Obesity are the top causes of a shortened life span ahead of diabetes, high blood pressure and high cholesterol, according to the latest statistics (*JAMA April 10, 2018*).

A previous report documented Obesity resulted in some 47% more life-years lost than tobacco, with tobacco as life-shortening as high blood pressure.

These results continue to highlight the importance of ceasing smoking, weight loss, diabetes management and healthy eating with diabetes, high blood pressure and high cholesterol all able to be treated.

These statistics are not age specific, which this book now does, but a guide as to what, over-all and long-term conditions, we should concentrate on minimising.

It can be seen these and all first world countries share the same Top 10.

The order will vary over the years but the "Top 10" are fairly constant.

TOP 10 CAUSES OF DEATH ALL AGES

	USA 2014	UK 2013	Australia 2015
1	Heart disease	Heart disease	Heart disease
2	Cancer	Lung cancer	Dementia Alzheimers
3	Ch low respiratory diseases	Dementia, Alzheimer's	Cerebrovascular disease
4	Unintentional injuries	Emphysema/bronchitis	Trachea, lung cancer
5	Cerebrovascular diseases	Cerebrovascular diseases	Chronic lower respiratory diseases
6	Alzheimer's D.	Flu/pneumonia	Diabetes
7	Diabetes mellitus	Prostate cancer	Colon cancer
8	Influenza, pneumonia	Bowel cancer	Blood, lymph cancer (leukaemia)
9	Kidney disease	Lymphoid cancer	Heart failure
10	Suicide	Liver disease	Diseases of the urinary system

SECTION B

HOW TO USE THE RELEVANT CHAPTER FOR YOUR AGE and SEX

The following chapters list the illnesses or risks that most occur for your present age and cause our premature deaths or disabilities.

Now aware of these you can take avoiding-preventive actions as documented. Then, it is recommended that you also look at the next decade to see how and what illnesses change and how to take preventive measures against those too.

Graphs show the individual proportion of deaths or disabilities.

ESSENTIAL
Just read the one chapter for your age:

- *Find the Chapter for your age and sex*
- See what serious illnesses occur
- Read how to avoid them

	Chapter	
	3	Overview
WOMEN	4	Young (5-19 UK; 15-24 USA)
	5	25 – 44 years
	5	45 – 64
	7	>65
MEN	8	< 24
	9	25 – 34 (44)
	10	45 – 64
	11	>65

RECOMMENDED
- Read the next Chapter
- See what future illnesses you are likely to encounter
- Take avoiding actions as recommended

DESIRABLE
The rest of the book is packed with beneficial health advice

TESTS and INVESTIGATIONS
- Relevant for your age

WOMEN
CAUSES OF PREMATURE DEATHS and DISABILITIES

For each age group

CHAPTER 3.
WOMEN: OVERVIEW

Womens' Greatest Concerns (UK)
1. Heart disease
2. Breast cancer
3. Osteoporosis
4. Depression
5. Autoimmune diseases

The following are the overall leading causes of Burden of Disease and Injury and should alert you to seek early help

Condition	% of Total
25 - 44 years	
Depression	12.1
Anxiety	6.2
Breast Cancer	4.9
Genito-urinary Diseases	4.2
Asthma	3.5
45 - 64 years	
Breast Cancer	10.0
Osteoarthritis	6.6
Ischemic Heart Disease	6.5
Diabetes mellitus	5.6
Depression	5.2
65 years and over	
Ischemic Heart Disease	20.3
Stroke	10.7
Alzheimer's / Dementia	8.9
Ch Obstructive Pulmonary Disease	4.0
Breast cancer	3.6

Note: These are conditions which make someone disabled and may or may not include the cause of death.

CHAPTER 4.
YOUNG WOMEN

Be aware – get help – get checked

USA Females 15 – 24 yrs	England and Wales 5 – 19 yrs
RTA	RTA*
Suicide	Suicide
Poisonings	Homicide
Homicide	Lymphoid Cancer
Endocrine Disorders	Congenital Defects
Other Injuries	Cerebral palsy
Congenital Anomalies	Brain Cancer
Maternal conditions	Accidental poisoning
Leukemia	Accidental breathing threats
Influenza / Pneumonia	Emphysema / Bronchitis

England and Wales figures are from age 5 years with more Infantile conditions.

For the 15 to 24 years old age group Road Accidents predominate then Suicide and this is where most emphasis needs to be placed.

Counselling not to drink and drive and to wear seat belts cannot be over emphasized or repeated enough.

Suicide watch is all important: Any mood changes, withdrawal, sadness, volatility or frank depression must be given immediate attention and intensive observation and support.

*RTA = Road Traffic Accidents

Live Longest Compendium   145

CHAPTER 5.

WOMEN AGED 25–44 YEARS

"Depression, Anxiety and Cancer"

Be aware – get help – get checked:

Causes of Female Deaths

	% USA 25 - 34	England-Wales 20 - 34	Australia 25 - 44
1	Unintentional Injuries 31.2	Poisoning	Suicide
2	Cancer 12.6	Accidental poisoning	Accidental poisoning
3	Suicide 9.3	RTA	RTA
4	Heart Dis 7.4	Breast Ca	CAD

Disabilities
As noted, Causes of Premature Death are not always in the same order as Causes of Premature Disabilities.

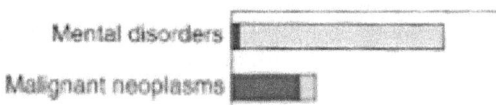

The light bar gives the proportion of Disabilities; the dark bar the amount of deaths. It can be seen how non-fatal (light bar) Mental Disorders far outstrip any deaths they may cause whereas the greatest cause of deaths are cancers (Malignant Neoplasms, mostly Breast Cancer- the dark bar).

Causes of Premature Deaths and Disabilities 25 - 44 yrs
Be aware – get help – get checked
1. Mental disorders (Disability far greater than Deaths)
2. Malignant neoplasms (cancer)
3. Chronic Respiratory Diseases
4. Genito-urinary diseases (100% disability - not fatal)
5. Musculoskeletal diseases (100% disabilities- not fatal)
6. Unintentional injuries
7. Cardiovascular disease
8. Intentional injuries (100% fatal - ?related to 1 Mental disorders)
9. Digestive system diseases
10. Nervous system disorders

Disability problems for this age group (25-44 years) are:

Mental illnesses
Depression 38%
Anxiety 33%

As a group the greatest cause of disabilities in this 25–44-year-old age group for women is dominated by mental disorders, which in turn are mainly due to depression (38%) and anxiety (33%) causing disability rather than deaths.

While deaths, according to this data set, are relatively few, it is to be noted that for "8. Intentional injuries", by which we can only assume suicide, deaths are 100%, and surely the result of a mental illness be it acute or chronic depression. All such young women must be watched like hawks. If it is yourself, you must seek both medical and social support.

Drugs or illicit substances do not seem to play as much a role as with young men, but the liberation of women may make this an impression rather than an actual fact. After all, women are smoking and drinking alcohol more, which usually shadows drug and substance abuse.

The explosion of hormones provides a roller coaster ride for many young women with unrealized and confused ambitions. Marrying your childhood sweetheart and having kids before the age of 20 is no longer the preferred career move. But what is? A world perceived to be male-dominated and offering less career satisfaction might frustrate, confuse and depress the more ambitious. Coping with the workplace and accepting responsibility can engender anxiety in those promoted beyond their experience. A turbulent home life exacerbates problems.

Most seem to settle in their 30s but the "Big 4-0" make some women sit up, look around and wonder if there isn't more to life and if it isn't passing them by.

While unpleasant, most of these mental disorders respond to treatment and do not account for many deaths.

It is my personal belief that there are too many antidepressants prescribed and most of any beneficial effect they may achieve is due to the placebo effect. Cognitive Behaviour Therapy- support – is to be preferred. With support, time will see improvements.

Cancer
Cancer accounts for 13% of the disabilities in this age group, of which breast cancer predominates at 37% and is the one of the greatest causes of death. Early diagnosis is essential.
What to do:
Mammograms, examinations and pap smears should be done.
Genetic counseling if there is a family history.

Chronic Respiratory Disease
This is essentially the same as the advice for men (above).

Genito-Urinary Disease
Sexually Transmitted Diseases (STD) are likely and increasing incredibly in the sexually active with multiple partners. Intercourse, childbirth and the anatomy where the opening of the urethra is so close to the vagina and anus make women much more susceptible to urinary tract infections. It is essential that these be completely cleared each time or there is the chance of chronic infection, which can then ascend to the kidney—a far greater problem. The gold standard is to get a mid-stream urine specimen to identify the germ, and the best antibiotic, and then repeat it after the course to make sure the urine is now sterile.

Childbirth can also distort the anatomy, making infections more easily acquired as well as causing the uterus to displace and incontinence.

Regular checks and pap smears are mandatory.

Musculoskeletal
Musculoskeletal disorders don't often cause death and include osteo and rheumatoid arthritis and chronic back pain. Back pain increases dramatically at age 20 years to 54, unlike the arthritides, which increase later at 40 years. There can be no doubt that it can be a severe problem. Often a cause cannot be found. Much can be prevented by strong core muscles (para-spinal and abdominal), being fit, reducing abdominal fat and avoiding unnatural postures especially while lifting.

Cardiovascular Disease (CVD)
CVD surprisingly manifests later in women or is under-diagnosed. Any undue fatigue, shortness of breath on exertion or chest pain must be investigated. Get BP checked regularly and an ECG/EKG if asymptomatic when you hit 40, your LDL at 30, as a baseline record.

Digestive Tract Disorders

Digestive system diseases run the spectrum from indigestion and cancer (covered above) to ulcers, irritable bowel syndrome, Crohn's Disease, ulcerative colitis and piles. Weight loss and tiredness are often the early symptoms, while the passing of blood or mucus is an early sign. Recurrent abdominal pain, swelling or diarrhea must be investigated.

Nervous System Disorders

Multiple Sclerosis or rare disorders occur at this age for which there are no prevention or treatments except for specialized rehab centers.

The following Graph shows the proportions of both Premature Deaths and Disabilities.

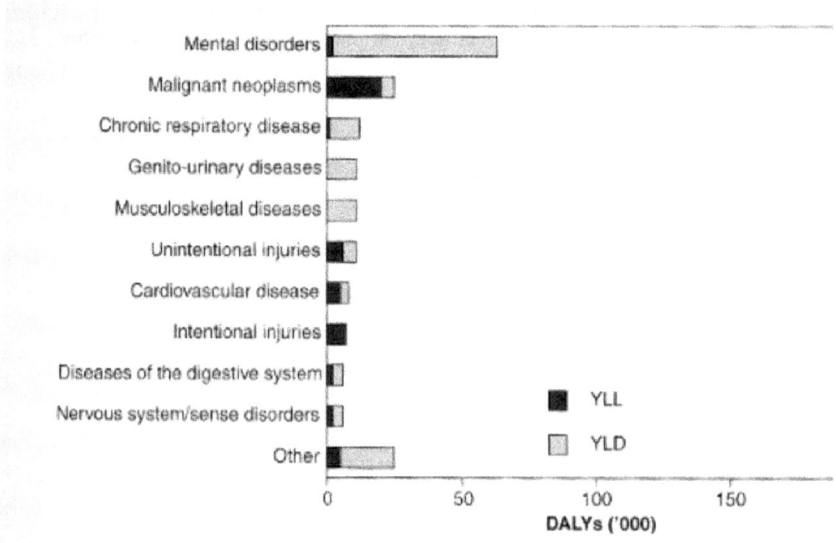

Source: Australian Burden of Disease and Injury Study.

Leading causes of burden of disease and injury in women aged 25–44 years

Light Bar = Premature Disabilitiy
Dark Bar = Premature Deaths

CHAPTER 6.
WOMEN AGED 45–64 YEARS

"Cancer (breast, lung, colon) and Heart "

Be aware – get help – get checked:

Causes of Premature Deaths

	% USA 45 - 54	England & Wales 35-49	Australia 45 -64
1	Cancer (Breast, Lung, CRC) 32.8	Breast Ca	CAD
2	Heart Disease 15.1	Liver D	Lung Ca
3	Unintentional injuries 9.7	Accidental poisoning	Breast Ca
4	Ch Liver D 4.2	Suicide	Suicide
5	Low Respiratory D 3.5	IHD	CRC

Causes of Premature Deaths and Disabilities
1. Malignant neoplasms (cancer) 13%
2. Cardiovascular disease 5.7%
3. Mental disorders (Disability far greater than deaths)
4. Musculoskeletal diseases (100% disabilities- not fatal)
5. Nervous system disorders
6. Chronic Respiratory Diseases
7. Diabetes mellitus
8. Unintentional injuries
9. Digestive system diseases
10. Oral health

This is quite a difference from the younger previous group wherein the dominant mental issues of Depression and Anxiety and Intentional injuries have been displaced by Cancer and Heart Disease and surprisingly no Genito-urinary issues - presumably addressed in the earlier sexually active and child-bearing age group. The Respiratory diseases are mostly due to smoking then asthma but Diabetes mellitus (Type 1 - insulin dependent) makes its first appearance while oral health makes its first and only appearance. Time to get your teeth fixed - pity about the lack of fluoride as a kid.

Problems for age 45–64 women:
This is the most dangerous age for breast cancer, but other cancers occur as well, while heart disease and strokes impact.

Cancer
    Breast cancer 30%
    Lung 14%
    Colorectal 13%.

Cardiovascular Disease 14%
    IHD 47%
    Strokes 29%

Mental Disorders
    Depression 51%.
    Anxiety 33%

Osteoarthritis 7%

Diabetes 6%
The cancer and cardiovascular disease are more often fatal, whereas the others more often result in non-fatal burdens.

Menopause
Varies from mild to severe. Duavive/Duovee is a combination product containing conjugated estrogens and bazedoxifene (an oestrogen agonist/antagonist). It is used by women with a uterus to help reduce symptoms of menopause and, in my experience, is superior to the usual HRT

What to do:
Breast Cancer
1 in 8 women will develop cancer of the breast.
Regular examinations by your doctor.
Learn to self-examine—you have more time than anyone else.
Regular mammograms. Mammograms are arguably the best screen test, but some 1 in 6 cancers are missed. Also have regular pap smears.

Lung Cancer
Get a chest x-ray or CT scan / MRI if coughing blood / losing weight
Lung cancer and COPD are invariably due to smoking tobacco or marijuana and are preventable. But be alert to any past workplace contaminants such as asbestos, which may be as "innocent" as lagging on factory or ships' pipes or on old roofs and walls.

Colorectal Cancer
Have a colonoscopy if any passage of blood or mucus.

Cardiovascular Disease
Ischemic heart disease means the blood supply to the heart is compromised by cholesterol plaques and narrowing of the coronary arteries This usually first manifests as heart pain on exertion (angina) and must be treated and monitored.
Report any chest pain or heat flutters—possible ECG/EKG
Also see note regarding aspirin in relevant men's' age group.

Strokes
Make sure you are on a low-dose pill.

Skin Cancer and Melanoma
Like all cancers they "take off" after the age of 40 and increase. This is due to excessive ultraviolet radiation—sun exposure. Like lung cancer it is not the one packet of cigarettes but the regular exposure to the carcinogens (smoke or sun) over some 20 years that initiates the mutation of the DNA in our cells to become cancers. Skin cancer can be seen, and therefore most can be diagnosed early enough to effect a cure. Get checked annually especially in sunbelt regions.

Mental Issues
Treat depression/anxiety. Cognitive Behavioral Therapy ? preferable to drugs.

By now suicide seems to not be the potential threat it is with younger women, so support is what was and probably is needed.

The average age for menopause is 53 and this comes as a psychological as well as hormonal insult. Here oestrogen is abruptly cut off. It is a violent hormonal change with no male equivalent but obviously can herald many mixed emotions.

Osteo Arthritis
My best analogy is that OA is "rust" in the joints. It can run the gamut from inconsequential to being completely debilitating.
Report any finger joint lumps, and hand, knee, or hip pain or stiffness.
Keeping mobile (like moving and using a rusty hinge) is all-important.

Diabetes

Get a Random Blood Glucose test.

As noted elsewhere, diabetes 2 is usually associated with being overweight, but I have some slim and fit diabetics in my practice, and some with no family history.

The first line of treatment is the *Newtrition Super-Mediterranean Diet (Book 2)*.

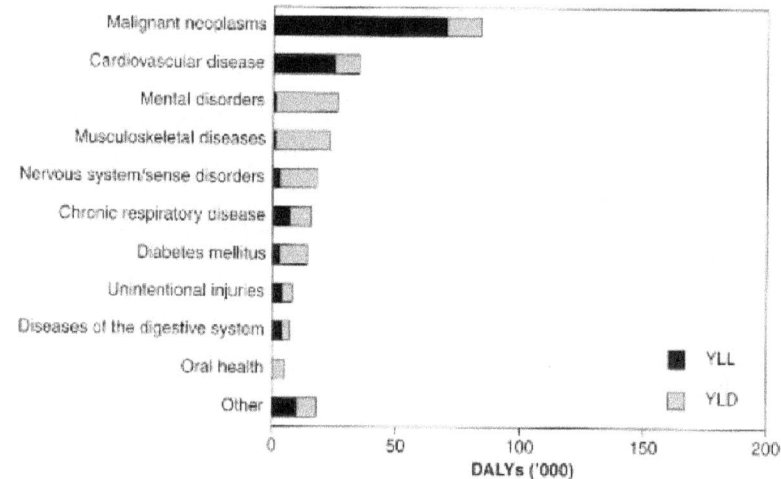

Source: Australian Burden of Disease and Injury Study.

Leading causes of burden of disease and injury in women aged 45-64 years

Dark band = Premature Deaths
Light band = Premature Disabilities

CHAPTER 7.
WOMEN 65 YEARS AND OVER

"Oh my (irregularly) Beating Heart"

Be aware – get help – get checked:

Causes of Premature Deaths and Disabilities in Order
1. Cardiovascular disease
2. Malignant neoplasms (cancer)
3. Nervous system disorders
4. Chronic Respiratory Diseases
5. Musculoskeletal diseases (100% disabilities - not fatal)
6. Diabetes mellitus
7. Digestive system diseases
8. Unintentional injuries
9. Genito-urinary diseases
10. Acute Respiratory diseases

The main health problems in older women are:

Cardiovascular 37.2%
IHD (heart) is the main cardiovascular problem at 54.4%, then stroke at 28.8%.

Cancer 20.8%
Colorectal cancer 16.4%
Breast 15.1%
Lung 15.1%.

Nervous system disorders 17.9%
Of which Alzheimer's / dementia 49.7%

Hearing and vision loss 32.1%

Parkinson's 12.2%

Acute Respiratory Infections

Cardiovascular problems now take over from cancer as the greatest cause of disabilities or problems.

Heart attacks and strokes present most problems: Blood Pressure, any heart arrhythmias and elevated LDL cholesterol and triglycerides must be checked and controlled. Achieve optimum weight and exercise (dancing is great).

Mental disorders have disappeared, and teeth have been fixed but regular six-monthly ultra-sound cleaning should be done. People with chronic gum disease are 20% to even 70% more likely to get dementia/Alzheimer's.

The early signs of Dementia manifest and Nervous System disorders, rare in the younger, such as Parkinson's Disease which manifests with increasingly small handwriting, frozen expression, shuffling and "pill rolling" tremors. Eyesight and hearing problems begin or worsen.

As noted previously, you are now "old," but as with the age-old saying, "You are only as old as you feel"; or, you can still have "joie de vivre"—the joy of life.

Get a dog, garden, learn a new skill (music, Sudoku, a language), socialize, have a purpose, be optimistic. All contribute to reduced cognitive decline and a longer life. **See Book 2 Successful Aging.**

I am continually amazed at people who groan as they undress and have to be helped onto the examination table and complain "It's awful getting old, doctor." They are slow, bent, dull and look old, many have no debilitating illnesses but their whole attitude is wrong.

It has recently been claimed that, "75 is the new 65"; and due to improved nutrition, public health measures and modern medicine this is indeed the case. So being "65 and over" does not condemn you to the retirement village but rather is a call to increase your pursuit of health and vitality. Be an optimist. There are a lot of people worse off. When I had whining introspective patients in hospital with not much wrong but who pestered us out of proportion to their ailment, I had them moved close to someone terminally ill and when that patient died, the change in the hypochondriacs was always startling. One of my "treatments" for bad sleep is to recommend the patient listen to the radio news. After the suicide bombings, refugee drownings, and the ghastly tsunami of bad news on bad news, the penny drops, and they (should) realise they don't have such horrors to contend with. Their anxiety over what was keeping them awake is not as great as these misfortunes; they (hopefully) gain some objectivity and they go to sleep. But, obviously, if this upsets you more, don't do it.

We all have to die, but the whole essence of this book is to live it up and stay healthy as long as you can. Don't become a premature invalid or prematurely old because of a bad mental attitude. At 65 and over there is the distinct danger of people winding down because that is how they think society is geared. Well, read *The New York Times* obituaries and see just how many were rock and rollin' into their 90s.

What to do:
- An ECG/EKG now mandatory to rule out atrial fibrillation and reduce strokes.
- Colon cancer has now overtaken breast cancer, so report any change of bowel habit, undue/unexplained fatigue or anemia, and chronic diarrhoea; consider a colonoscopy.
- Continue mammograms and breast examinations.
- Report any ongoing coughs.
- Get a chest x-ray if there is past history of smoking.
- Staying fit with mental challenges is all-important. Alzheimer's and Parkinson's, while inevitable, can be remarkably delayed by doing so. Even ballroom dancing and bridge helps.
- Get eyes and hearing checked.
- Report any tremors, shuffling, smaller writing.
- Get any chest infections treated aggressively and promptly. Review and do annually.
- Get skin checked more regularly if damaged and living in a sunbelt zone and while, in the 1920s, Coco Chanel made us admire and desire a tan where previously it was a marker of outdoor peasants, there is no such thing as a 'safe' tan.
- Get the flu shot.

Many of these deaths and disabilities may seem sudden, like a heart attack or a stroke; but in truth, most have been brewing and incubating for decades. If we are at our healthiest at age 11, then by 40 years our tests reveal a sudden spurt of bad results. Most of these we don't notice. Our raised blood pressure and blood lipids are asymptomatic; we may be more thirsty and void more from diabetes, but the joint pains are usually mild and just starting, and any symptoms of cancer are not usually flagrant—perhaps a little tiredness, usually passed off. And so, most usually from self-inflicted abuse of high-risk behaviors, we have spent three decades, from 10 to 40 years of age, accumulating damage. The only outside signs are overweight/obesity and the only one we notice is pushing the paper farther away to read.

Perhaps life doesn't begin at 40.

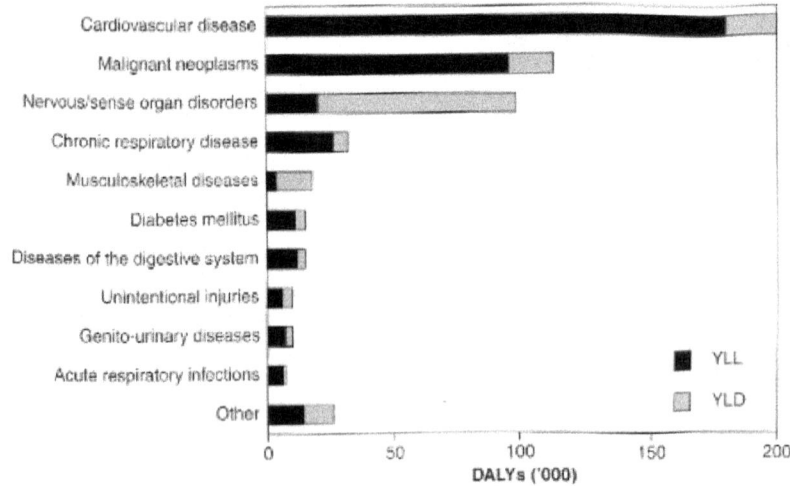

Leading causes of burden of disease and injury in women aged 65 years and over

Light bar = **YLD** = "Healthy" **Years Lost due to Disability** = Non-fatal burden of illness

Dark bar = **YLL** = **Years of Life Lost** due to premature death by the same illness

DALY = YLL + YLD = Total Burden

One DALY is the equivalent of one year of healthy life lost.

MEN

CAUSES OF PREMATURE DEATHS and DISABILITIES

For each age group

CHAPTER 8.
MEN UNDER 24 YEARS

Be aware – get help – get checked:

USA Males 20-24	UK Males 5 - 19 yrs	Australia 15-24
Unintentional injuries 42.7%	Transport Accidents (Land)	Suicide
Suicide 18.8%	Suicide	Motor Accidents
Homicide 16.8%	Homicide	Accidental Poisoning
Cancer 4.2%	Lymphoid Cancer	Assault
Heart Disease 3.0%	Congenital Defects	Undetermined events
Birth Defects 0.8%	Cerebral Palsy/Syndromes	
Diabetes 0.6%	Brain Cancer	
Flu & Pneumonia 0.5%	Accidental Poisoning	
Ch Lower Respiratory D	Accidental breath threats	
Stroke 0.5%	Emphysema / Bronchitis	

Suicide and accidents, especially, vehicle accidents top the lists in all countries.

High-risk behavior is common in young men and leads to injuries and deaths, but the data on "fun activities" is not well known e.g. youth and adolescents 5–19 years of age who were treated in US emergency departments an average of 176 a day for skateboarding-related injuries. While these mostly do not cause death, the risks are underestimated and dangerous. Quad bikes are the greatest cause of injury and deaths on farms. Diving into shallow water, drugs, alcohol and driving too fast are perhaps better known.

What to do:
In the next age group "Drugs, Booze and Testosterone" are manifesting. It is a too-often deadly combination as youth experiments and pushes the boundaries.

Parental control can give way to guidance and advice, but this age group consider themselves "bullet proof" and only the death of a close friend may alert them to modify their high-risk behaviors.

Sport is the traditional outlet to attenuate the aggression that testosterone brings but any contact-sport head injury, even mild, results in long-term brain damage.

Suicide figures prominently and any signs of with-drawl, depression or "problems" must be acted on urgently.

Homicide would seem inexorably linked to liberal gun laws.

Drugs: Finally, I have so many nice, well balanced, hard-working patients in my practice who, much to my surprise, contracted Hepatitis C, which means they were injecting illicit drugs when young. They are all embarrassed and sheepish about it now and thank goodness Hep C is now curable. And while they all claim they regret it, and wouldn't do it again, the temptation must have been so great that even these ostensibly well-adjusted people were tempted to try drugs.

Just don't. They all have long term damage.

Tattoos: Tatts are as old as the world and usually symbolic of tribal culture. Fashion goes in vogues and today, most young people are encouraged to join the crowd and get a Tat ...and then another.

It is, however, a universal regret when they reach middle or old age and what may have seemed exciting and fashionable in one's 20s is now rather embarrassing and pathetic in one's 50s.

Resist the temptation and see if you still want one when you are 50.

CHAPTER 9.
MEN 25–34 (44) YEARS

"Drugs, Booze and Testosterone"

Drugs, booze and testosterone account for 70% of all deaths and disabilities in this age group, which is where to focus.

Be aware – get help – get checked:

CAUSES OF DEATHS

USA 25 - 34 yrs	UK 20 - 34 yrs	Australia 25 - 44
1 RTA	Suicide	Suicide
2 Homocide	Accidental Poisoning	Accidents
3 Suicide	RTA	Cancer
4 Poisoning	Homocide	Cardiovascular Disease
5 Other Injuries	Liver Disease	Infections / Parasitic
6 Drownings	Epilepsy	Mental Disorders
7 Endocrine Disorders	Heart Disease	Others
8 Congenital Abnormalities	Brain Cancer	Nervous Disorders
9 Inflammatory / Heart	Lynphoid Cancer	Digestive disorders
10 Leukemia	Cerebrovascular Disease	Ch Respiratory Disease

EVIDENCED PREVALENCE	PREVENTIVE MEASURES
1. Drugs & Booze – 38% Depression	Consider all males in this age group as substance abusers until proven otherwise. Warn and advise. Watch for depression—suicide.
2. Homicide (USA / UK)	Access to guns is the problem.
3. RTA / Accidents – 15%	Fast cars, testosterone and booze. Advice, counseling Motor Bikes: 5% of vehicles but 25% of MVAs.
4. Suicide – 12%	Heightened awareness that this age group is at risk. Early diagnosis, support, advice
5. Cancer	Smoking and processed foods promote Change of bowel habit, smoker's cough
6. CVS	Shortness of breath on effort, chest pain. Screen.
7. Infections	Cause. Overseas travel prophylaxis.
8. Chronic Respiratory Diseases	Asthma/emphysema. Cease smoking
9. Musculoskeletal Diseases – Back Pain	Back pain starts at 20. Lifting advice
10. Nervous Sys Multiple Sclerosis	No preventive measures as yet.
11. Digestive System	Heartburn: Lose weight, stop smoking, reduce booze, avoid PPIs.

As a group the greatest cause of disabilities in this 25–44-year-old age group for men is **mental disorders,** which in turn are mainly due to **substance abuse—alcohol and illicit drugs (38%)** and **depression (27%)** causing disability rather than premature deaths. Knowing that drugs, substance abuse and depression cause so many problems may facilitate an earlier diagnosis. Getting on the front foot and aggressively treating rather than suspecting depression is also arguably warranted. All illicit drugs cause damage. The opioid epidemic in the USA is a major problem.

Unintentional Injuries are second and *contribute more to death than disabilities* (as do the next five causes). They account for 15.5%, of which almost half are from road traffic accidents (RTA). This group represents the testosterone-fueled, high-risk behavior group—smoking, drinking, "never thinking of tomorrow," experimenting, showing off, driving too fast. Dietary advice should have started as well. Motorbikes account for 5% of vehicles but 25% of accidents. Skate Boards and Mountain Biking take an increasing toll.

Intentional Injuries come third, making up some 12% of the total. Breaking down such injuries, 85% are due to suicide or self-inflicted injuries.

However, the largest *single* cause of disease and injury burden in this age group is suicide and self-inflicted injuries, at 10.3%; then depression (7.4%), road traffic accidents (6.6%), alcohol dependence/misuse (5.8%), HIV/AIDS (4.5%).

The message here is to get on the front foot and proactively assume depression and offer support, intervention and treatment to prevent suicide or attempted suicide. This, I feel, cannot be over-emphasized.

In the United States, due to their liberal gun laws, homicide is high on the list; but it is high also in the United Kingdom.

Knifings are an increasing UK problem.

Cancer or malignant neoplasms are next, with brain cancers more common than most of us think; these are invariably fatal. Again, early diagnosis offers the best hope. Watch for any change of behavior. Cancer of the colon (CAC) is another we don't really associate with young men, but there are some famous young widows whose husbands died from CAC. Unexplained loss of weight, change of bowel habit, passing mucus, slime or blood, and undue fatigue are symptoms and signs.

Cardiovascular disease usually manifests later, but any undue fatigue or shortness of breath on exertion must be investigated. While the annual physical has been found a pretty useless ritual, getting one each decade in your 20s and 30s would seem warranted to listen for heart murmurs, EC/KG abnormalities and lipids. In this age group congenital abnormalities are more to be found than those caused by poor diet.

Infectious and parasitic diseases are usually communicable diseases spread by bacteria or viruses by airborne droplets, insects, and contaminated food; or, they are sexually transmitted. Everyone should be vaccinated against as many illnesses as possible. After that, continue to take care of personal hygiene.

Chronic Respiratory Disease is invariably the result of smoking, either active or passive, tobacco or marijuana and, as such, is preventable. Asthma is also an underestimated chronic illness where research reveals sufferers under-treat themselves. Neglecting regular prevention medication and only seeking immediate emergency relief leads to unnecessary hospitalizations and even deaths. Again, a very preventable illness.

Musculoskeletal Diseases in these statistics don't cause death. They include osteo and rheumatoid arthritis, chronic back pain and even gout, all of which are popularly considered as occurring in the older populace. Back pain increases dramatically at age 20 years (to 54), unlike the arthritides, which increase later at 40 years. There can be no doubt that these conditions can be a severe problem, ever since "man became the only animal with enough arrogance to walk upright on his hind legs." Often a cause cannot be found, and this has led to abuse of the welfare system and a complicated psychiatric roundabout of "pain" gets reward." Much can be prevented by strong core muscles (para-spinal and abdominal), being fit, reducing abdominal fat and avoiding unnatural postures especially while lifting (bend the knees). Back surgery has improved by leaps and bounds.

Nervous System Disorders: At this age these cases are usually epilepsy or multiple sclerosis. Unfortunately, there are no prevention methods except for avoiding traumas that cause epilepsy.

Digestive System Diseases run the spectrum from indigestion to cancer (covered above), and include ulcers, irritable bowel syndrome, Crohn's disease, ulcerative colitis and piles.

Looking ahead, there is a dramatic change after 45, when heart disease and cancer raise their ugly heads. This fact should alert all to cease smoking and eat the *Newtrition Super-Mediterranen Diet (Book 1)*. The most obvious, and therefore frequently the most overlooked deduction, is that heart disease and cancer *don't* suddenly start at 45. If males do manage to live through their high-risk behavior years, avoiding unintentional or intentional injuries and substance abuse, they have, however, *not avoided causing the pathology that will kill or burden them.* As well as addressing these high-risk behaviors by being alert to possible depression and potential suicide, we should also be looking at what prevents the diseases that manifest after 45.

You will also see that mental illness and suicide dramatically decrease with age. It would be more than cynical to suggest that this is because all the fragile males have already topped themselves. Rather it is the accepted medical wisdom that if we can get them through these high-risk years, their mental state stabilizes to normal, so it's worth being aware and making the effort.

Hearing loss intrudes after 40. Stop exposure to loud noise now.

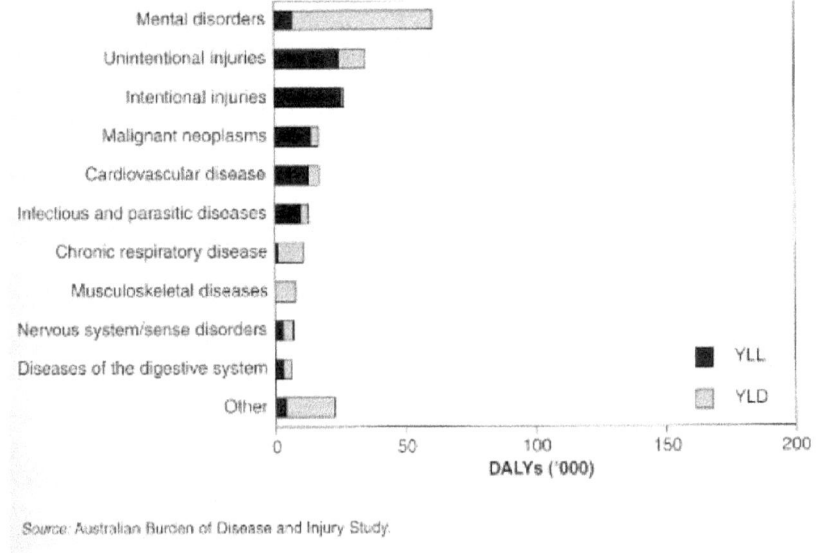

Leading causes of burden of disease and injury in men aged 25-44 years

Light Bar = Premature Disabilities (YLD)
Dark Bar = Premature Deaths (YLL)
DALY = Years lost to both.

CHAPTER 10.
MEN 35-44-64 YEARS

"The Male Menopause, Heart Attacks and Cancer"

Overall
The drugs, booze, smoking, junk food, being overweight and unfit have now caught up and cardiovascular disease and cancer affect over half of these men. Look ahead at what illnesses are most likely when over 65. These are what you must now try to prevent, as well as getting early diagnosis of any current ailments (CardioVascularDisease increases significantly at 65 but cancer does not).

Be aware – avoid these - get help – get checked:

Causes of Deaths

	USA 35 - 44 years	UK 35 - 49	Australia 45 - 64
1	Suicide	Suicide	CVD
2	Poisoning	Heart Disease	Cancer
3	CAD	Liver Disease	Accidents
4	RTA	Accidental Poisoning	Digestive D
5	Homicide	CVD	Ch Lung D
6	Liver Disease	Lung Cancer	Diabetes mellitus
7	Hypertension	RTA	Nervous Syst
8	Diabetes mellitus	CAC	Mental
9	CVA	Lymphoid Cancer	Genito-urinary
10	CAC	Brain Cancer	Musculoskeletal

CAD = Coronary Artery Disease. CVD = Coronary Vascular Disease (essentially the same)
RTA = Road Traffic Accidents
CAC = Cancer of the Colon

Causes of Premature Deaths and Disabilities in Order 45-64
1. Cardiovascular disease
2. Malignant neoplasms (cancer)
3. Nervous system disorders
4. Mental disorders (Disability far greater than deaths)
5. Chronic Respiratory Diseases
6. Diabetes mellitus
7. Unintentional injuries
8. Musculoskeletal diseases (100% disabilities)
9. Digestive system diseases
10. Genito-urinary diseases
11. Other

Disabling conditions most affecting 45–64-year-old males:
1. Ischemic heart disease 17%
2. Lung cancer 7%
3. Nervous system 7%
4. Mental disorders 6%
5. COPD (Chronic Obstructive Pulmonary Disease) 5%
6. Diabetes 5%
7. Hearing Loss 5%

Causes of disease and injury burden: Men aged 45–64
1. Cardiovascular disease 26%
2. Ischemic Heart Disease 64%
3. Strokes 17%
4. Cancer 25%
5. Lung 26%
6. Colorectal 16%

What to do:
Get help if depressed or if any suicidal thoughts
At 35 or 40 it is time to get a base-line level for all medical tests as per Section 4: Tests and Diagnoses.
But especially: Get BP, lipids, BG, Liver Function Tests and CXR done
Immediately stop smoking
Adopt *Newtrition Super-Mediterranean Foods (Book 1)*
Consider low-dose aspirin twice a week to help prevent stomach and colon cancer (needs 10 years and side effects, mostly bleeding, not now really recommended)
Get fit
Report wheeze, difficult breathing, chronic cough, bloody phlegm
Get a hearing test if any difficulties.

Suicide

It is a surprise that suicide is the number one killer for men aged 35 to 50 years in the USA and England/Wales. One can only conjecture as to the causes, Unfulfilled ambitions, failed love, business failure, the Global Financial crash, the Male Menopause, but psychiatry for too long has got bogged down as to aetiology (cause) and not got on with treatment - rather like asking someone bleeding to death from a leg wound 'how it happened' rather than staunching the loss and applying a tourniquet.

A little-known fact is that it is not known how anti-depressants work and that the only reliable anti-depressant over the last 25 years is called Placebo.

All are at risk and the best help is support from all sources, family, health workers, friends, social groups. Any talk of suicide, even a seeming joke, is a red-flag emergency.

Cardiovascular disease

Ischemic Heart Disease means the blood supply to the heart is compromised by cholesterol plaques and narrowing of the coronary (heart) arteries. This usually first manifests as heart Central chest, indigestion-like pain on exertion (angina) and must be treated and monitored. Any chest pain, undue fatigue or shortness of breath on exertion must be investigated. It would be advisable to get your blood pressure checked, to listen for heart murmurs, and ECG/EKG and lipids (LDL) at ages 35, 45, 55 and 65.

Immediately report any transient weakness, loss of movement/coordination or vision.

Cancer

This age group, between 35 and 64, is where cancer is most likely and early diagnosis affords the best chances of cure or survival. Be aware of the early symptoms and signs. Report any cough, loss of weight, altered bowel habit, passing or coughing blood or mucus.

Cancer of the colon (CAC/CRC): Unexplained fatigue, loss of weight, change of bowel habit, and passing mucus, slime or blood are symptoms and signs. Get a blood test, and if slightly anemic get a colonoscopy. Fecal blood tests may pick up some, but colonoscopy is the gold standard. People who took an aspirin tablet (325 or 81 mg) at least twice a week (usually for headache or muscle pain) had a lower incidence of gastrointestinal tract cancers, especially colorectal cancers but it takes 10 years and the side effects of bleeding are such that it is now only recommended in some high-risk adults in their 50s and 60s. But it is now no longer recommended for primary prevention.

There is, however, a worrying increase in CAC in those under 50 years. It is imperative to stop any preserved meats (sausages, bacon, ham). One strip of ham per day increases the risk of CAC by 19%. Reduce all red meat to smaller helpings only twice a week. Alcohol also raises the risk of CAC while fibre form wholemeal bread and cereals/grains lowered it.

Lung cancer and COPD are invariably due to smoking tobacco or marijuana and are preventable. But be alert to any past workplace contaminants such as asbestos, which may be as "innocent" as lagging on factory or ships' pipes. If you are a smoker you must get regular chest x-rays. If you have a cough that hangs on, also get a chest x-ray. Better still, stop smoking.

Skin Cancer and Melanoma: Like all cancers they "take off" after the age of 40 and increase. This is due to excessive ultraviolet radiation—sun exposure. Like lung cancer it is not the one packet of cigarettes but the regular exposure to the carcinogens (smoke or sun) over some 20 years that initiates the mutation of the DNA in our cells to become cancers. The best feature of skin cancer is that it can be seen and therefore most can be diagnosed early enough to effect a cure. Get checked annually.

Nervous System Disorders: At this age these are multiple sclerosis or more, rare degenerative disorders, for which there are no prevention or treatments except for specialized rehab centers. Report any unexplained limb weakness, incoordination, vision disturbances, altered sensations, headaches.

Mental Problems: Usually anxiety or depression. Initially try cognitive behavioral therapy. Get help.

The "Male Menopause" is also a real entity, where the man feels he is losing his youthful vitality *("The Death of a Salesman"*) and may then seek to recreate it with a sports car and trophy mistress. While this may be an object of derision, it has been pointed out that monogamy is unnatural to most species and humans by living much longer have not been "prepared" by evolution for the long monogamous relationships that our new longevity provides. It is a subject too complex to deal with here, but an equitable divorce is better than a poisonous marriage. The ultimate objective being the welfare and prosperity of all concerned.

Asthma and emphysema are also very "underestimated" chronic illnesses where research shows sufferers under-treat themselves, especially as to regular prevention medication rather than immediate emergency relief leading to unnecessary hospitalizations and even deaths. Again, a very preventable illness.

Diabetes 2 (TD2) we associate with being fat but there are some skinny diabetics. Get a Blood Glucose test. If overweight with TD2 losing 15kg can fix it.

Musculoskeletal Diseases in these statistics don't cause death. They include osteo and rheumatoid arthritis, chronic back pain and even gout.

Back pain increases dramatically at age 20 years to 54, unlike the arthritides, which increase later at 40 years. There can be no doubt that it can be a severe problem ever since "man became the only animal with enough arrogance to walk upright on his hind legs." Often a cause cannot be found, and this has led to abuse of the welfare system and a complicated psychiatric roundabout of "pain" gets reward." Much can be prevented by strong core muscles (para-spinal and abdominal), being fit, reducing abdominal fat and avoiding unnatural postures especially while lifting. Getting a diagnosis allows for the most appropriate treatment. Physiotherapy, weight loss and having fit muscles, while maintaining flexibility and movement, are all important while using the minimum of analgesics. NSAIDS used as anti-inflammatories, while effective, cause heart attacks and I try to avoid them. There is a pecking order as to cardio toxicity, with Naprosyn being the least toxic.

If it persists a Magnetic Resonance Image (MRI) is mandatory for a diagnosis.

Digestive System Diseases: These run the spectrum from indigestion to cancer (covered above) to ulcers, irritable bowel syndrome, Crohn's Disease, ulcerative colitis and piles. Weight loss and tiredness are often the early symptoms, and the passing of blood or mucus is an early sign.

Genito-urinary: This usually means "prostate trouble," or Benign Prostate Hypertrophy (BPH) where the prostate enlarges, then pushes into the bladder causing frequent urination and nocturia—having to get up at night to void. There are drugs available, but one type causes feminizing side effects and reduced libido or performance. An interesting alternative may be one of the erection enhancers—Tadalafil (Cialis)—which in smaller doses relaxes the bladder's small muscle wall and relieves the nocturia. Bladder and kidney cancers are not unknown—report passing any pink-blood urine.

The usual treatment is a TURP - Trans Urethral Resection of the Prostate which is a rather brutal "re-bore' of the penis. Some advanced Radiology Departments offer Prostate Artery Embolization (PAE) with less risk, less pain, and less recovery time than traditional surgery. A new treatment in London offers steam treatment which reputedly takes only 15 minutes and gets good results.

Hearing loss: it is most important you become aware as to any reduction in your hearing. While there are different types, most are caused by exposure to loud noise (amplified music, machinery). Reduce exposure. Use earmuffs if using noisy machines. Turn TV and radio down.

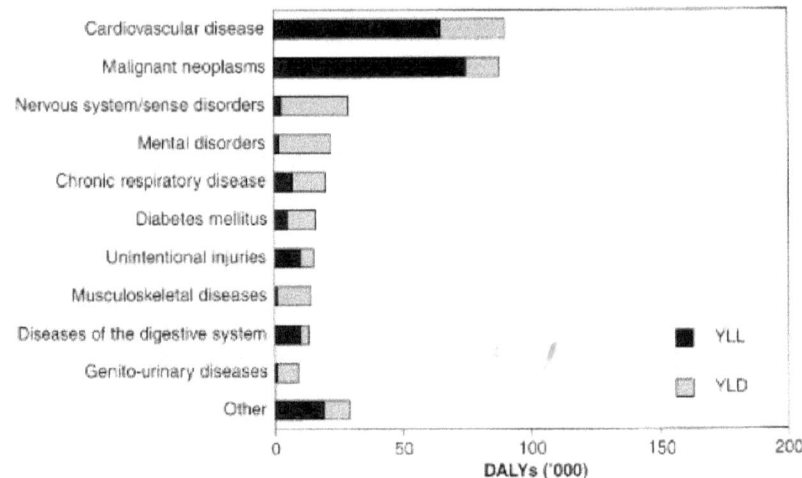

Source: Australian Burden of Disease and Injury Study.

Leading causes of burden of disease and injury in men aged 45–64 years

CHAPTER 11.
MEN 65 YEARS AND OVER

No mental issues: More Fatal Heart Attacks & Cancer

Be aware – avoid these - get help – get checked:

Causes of Deaths and for Australia Disabilities as well

	USA 65 years+	UK 65+	Australia 65+
1	CAD	IHD	CVD
2	Lung Disease	Cancer Lung	Cancer
3	Diabetes	Low Respiratory D	Nervous System
4	Stroke	CVD	Ch Lung D
5	Homicide	Ca Prostate	Genito-urinary
6	Cancer Colon		Diabetes mellitus
7	Hypertension		Digestive D
8	Cancer Pancreas		Musculoskeletal
9	Liver Cancer		Accidents
10			Endocrine/Metabolic

Cardiovascular disease has increased from 26% to 36% (i.e., more than a third), which makes it priority number one. Cancer has only increased by some 2% but it is still one of the major problems. At last, suicide is no longer high on the list.

You are now "old" as seen by those 30 years younger; but as Groucho Mark observed, "You are only as old as the woman you feel," which one observer interpreted as "proving it is never too late to find love."

I am continually amazed at old people who groan as they undress and have to be helped onto the examination table and complain, "It's awful getting old, doctor, wait till you're my age." They are slow, bent, dull and look old. They often have no debilitating illnesses but their whole attitude is wrong.

Someone recently said "75 is the new 65"; and due to improved nutrition, public health measures and modern medicine this is indeed the case. So being "65 and over" does not condemn you to the retirement village—rather it is a call to increase your pursuit of health and vitality. Be an optimist. There are a lot of people worse off. When I had whining introspective patients in hospital with not much wrong but who pestered us out of proportion to their ailment, I had them moved beside someone terminally ill; and when that patient died, the change in these hypochondriacs was always startling. One of my "treatments" for bad sleep is to recommend the patient listen to the radio news. Then after the suicide bombings, refugee drownings, and the ghastly tsunami of bad news upon bad news, the penny hopefully drops, and they realize they don't have such horrors to contend with. Their anxiety which was keeping them awake is not as great as these life-and-death struggles; with this new-found objectivity they can go to sleep. But more, this new-found perspective can and should be applied to every-day living. Carpe diem. If, however, it distresses youy more then Obviously discontinue.

We all have to die despite Silicon Valley's efforts, but the whole essence of this book is to live it up as long as you can. Don't become a premature invalid. At 65 and over there is the distinct danger of people winding down because that is how they think society is geared. Well, read *The New York Times* obituaries and see just how many were rock n rollin' into their 90s.

Cardiovascular Disease
Cardiovascular disease is mostly IHD (60%).
Strokes have risen from 17% to 24%.
This is where to place greatest priority
What to do:
Don't smoke
Report any chest pain, shortness of breath, ankle swelling
Get BP, LDL and BG checked
Get an ECG/EKG to exclude silent atrial fibrillation which is a major cause of strokes and now an epidemic for those over 60 years
Learn to feel your own pulse and if thready and irregular, get another ECG/EKG. AF can strike at any time and causes an irregular pulse.
An abdominal ultrasound is recommended to exclude an aortic aneurysm.
Adopt *Newtrition PHYTO Diet (Book 2)*, Successful Aging, Exercise and Weight programs (lose weight, cope with stress, challenge the brain).

Cancer
Lung cancer accounts for 26%. Stop smoking.
Prostrate 19%
Colorectal cancer 14%
Skin: get checked annually—more if in a sunbelt area.
What to do:
Get a chest x-ray
Report any urgency, frequency of urination or nocturia (having to get up at nights to void).

Report any alteration of bowel habit, passage of blood, mucus.
There are no satisfactory tests for cancer of the prostate, and in any event, it is often so slow growing, men die from something else. It is alleged that every male over 90 has cancer of the prostate.
Consider a colonoscopy. Cancer of the colon is curable detected early.

Nervous System Disorders
Alzheimer's/Dementia may begin. Be alert to signs
It is now more important than ever to accept new challenges and force the brain along and adopt the Newtrition Super-Mediterranean Diet.

The Rest
Follow the previous age group. Refer to the above but there is now greater urgency not to ignore what you may consider "minor" symptoms—as can be seen in the patient analysis of "Types" it is the proactive patient who achieves the best results for their health.
Stay fit, slim and active with plenty of new mental challenges.
Finally, see the chapter for age-specific tests and investigations.

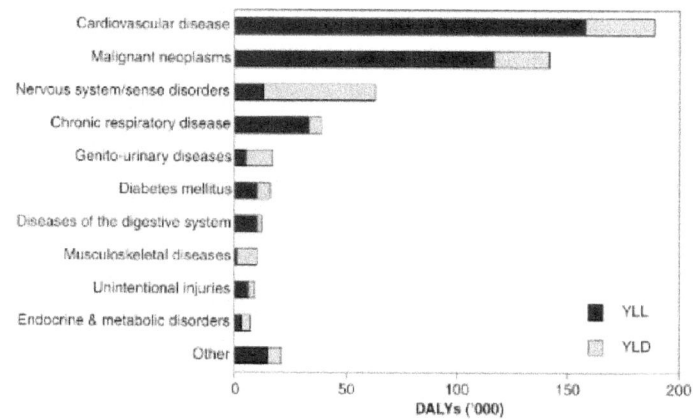

Leading causes of burden of disease and injury in men aged 65 years and over

Light bar = **YLD** = "Healthy" **Years Lost due to Disability** = Non-fatal burden of illness
Dark bar = **YLL** = **Years of Life Lost** due to premature death by the same illness
DALY = YLL + YLD = Total Burden
One DALY is the equivalent of one year of healthy life lost.

SECTION C

CHAPTER 12.
THE MISSING KEYS: RATIONALE

> Only 8% of us get correct Preventive advice
> Medical care prevents only 10% of premature deaths
> Healthy behaviours and lifestyle can improve this to 65%
> The Live Longest Preventive Advice may improve this to 90%
> It uniquely identifies the risks for your age & how to avoid them

The Missing Keys are the risks and illnesses identifying **WHAT'S GOING TO KILL YOU THIS YEAR so as to Live Longer Healthier.**

The corollary is Whamo! A surprise fatal illness or disability: *'It came out of left field'*, *'It was so unexpected'*, *'it was a complete shock'*, *'he looked so fit and healthy'*, *'(s)he just had the annual physical and all was well'*... and so on and on.

While we can't avoid all such surprise illnesses, now, for the first time, we can be fully aware of what risks and illnesses may await us and if you know which are likely to occur, then you can take special avoiding actions.

To date, however, it has been 'one size fits all' – the same annual medical checks and tests regardless of age and, guess what? They have been found next to useless: A review of 14 clinical trials and 182,000 patients followed for 9 years found that well patients derived no benefit from an annual physical exam.

By contrast, the Missing Keys as to What is Going to Kill You This Year now provides the best health information and advice relevant to your age and sex which, as flagged, this approach has until now been 'missing'.

Illness and chronic diseases are a tremendous burden causing premature death or disability...***but they are preventable in many instances.***

Yet only 8% of adults aged 35 or older received all recommended, high-priority, appropriate clinical preventive services, and nearly 5% received none.

These study figures are for Americans but applicable to most first world nations.

But what is staggering, a later survey found:

"Healthcare accounts for (only) between 5% and 15% (roughly 10%) of variation in premature death, whereas behavioural and social factors account for 16% to 65%".

This means that you are most likely to be one of the 92% to 95% who have not received such preventive advice and, your regular health checks account for only 10% to prevent you dying early or living in misery with a disability with, on average at age 60, one to three chronic diseases.

Or, to put it more clearly, up to two-thirds of our living longer-healthier is due to (healthy) behaviours or lifestyle, and not medical care.

It's what *you* can now do. You now have the choice to adopt the researched lifestyle(s) to live longer, longest, healthiest.

Living longer can be further improved, perhaps to 90%, by identifying and then avoiding the illnesses that hit us at certain ages. These are the Missing Keys.

And that is what this book now does: It informs you how and what to do.

Live Longer Healthier now provides you with this essential preventive advice to avoid premature death and disabilities, but more than this, tailors it to your present age and sex... **The Missing Keys as to WHAT'S GOING TO KILL YOU THIS YEAR**

Recent surveys have found:
- Some 60% of adults had at least one chronic disease or condition, and 42% had multiple diseases.
- Chronic diseases, including heart disease, cancer, chronic lung disease, stroke, Alzheimer's, diabetes, osteoarthritis, and chronic kidney disease, are the leading causes of poor health, long-term disability, and death.
- One-third of all deaths are attributable to heart disease or stroke, and every year, more than 1.7 million people receive a diagnosis of cancer.
- During the past several decades, the prevalence of diabetes increased dramatically.
- Diabetes increases the risk of developing other chronic diseases.
- Heart attack rates were on the decline but are now increasing surprisingly in adults in their 20s and 30s.

Chronic diseases profoundly reduce quality of life for patients and for their families, affecting enjoyment of life, family relationships, and finances. Working can be difficult. Functional limitations can be distressing, and depression, which can reduce a patient›s ability to cope with pain and worsen the clinical course of disease, is a common complication.

Chronic diseases are also the leading drivers of health care costs with diabetes, Alzheimer›s, and osteoarthritis being the most expensive.

Around 12% of the preventable harm was severe (causing prolonged, permanent disability or death), while incidents relating to drugs and other treatments accounted for almost half (49%) of preventable harm.

Clinical preventive strategies combined with lifestyle changes as recommended in this book, can substantially reduce the incidence of chronic disease and premature disability and death associated with chronic disease.

CHAPTER 13.

HOW TO BEST USE THESE LISTS
and Further Helpful Information

PREDICT and PREVENT the illnesses that occur for your age.

You really only need the one chapter appropriate to your age.
- Find the Section for your sex, then the Chapter for your age
- See what serious illnesses occur
- Read how to avoid them

Then
- Read the next Chapter
- See what illnesses you are likely to encounter in the future
- Take avoiding action

However,
A. PREMATURE DEATH
1. *Read the General Top 10 causes of death* so as to get the long-term perspective e.g. heart or cardiovascular disease is our greatest killer but in our 20s we are bullet-proof, and no one has a heart attack (but we are laying down the foundations for one and other fatal illnesses). So, understanding the long-term risks allows us to adopt the healthiest lifestyles *now* to prevent the long-term damage.

2. *Then find the Specific Causes chapter for your sex and age group*
This identifies those illnesses of greater incidence and risk for your age. And then read what to do.

3. *Finally, read the next age group chapter*
This will identify the illnesses most likely to be next, so you can reinforce preventive measures against those too.

B. PREMATURE DISABILITIES
If you don't die from a serious illness you are invariably disabled but more than this, are the insidious onset of disabling impositions we don't recognise as such, like deafness, until it's too late.

We are experiencing the "Diseases of Affluence" because we are now the richest society civilisation has ever witnessed. We have processed food available 24 hours a day, seven days a week, we have cars or public transport, labour saving devices, so we don't walk, garden, mow or eat fresh produce. It irks us to get up from the sofa to find the remote-control. In other words, we have become more sedentary, less physical and have a worse diet. And I am talking about day to day activities which therefore accumulate.
The end result is that we are the fattest humans ever. And getting fatter.

The USA, UK and Cuba were never healthier than with the great dust-bowl depression, World War 2 and the USA Economic Sanctions of Cuba. These restricted and rationed food and imposed exercise (no petrol).

We are now chronically over-eating and over-eating unnatural, factory additive foods and under-exercising. Yet the longest living people grow and eat their own vegetables – not only exercising, by gardening, but eating what evidence suggests is the food group most beneficial to our health – vegetables.

I have detailed what to eat in Book 2 NEWTRITION - which is my updated, improved "SUPER-Mediterranean Diet". The WHO has stated that the Mediterranean Diet is the healthiest and I have updated and upgraded it to "Super" status.

While we are living longer we seem to be carrying more disabilities. Most, if not all, patients I see, who are over 60, are on some medication. Some are on 10 or more! Yet the incredible advances in public health – a pure water supply, vaccinations, hygiene, disease control, better nutrition – should and *could* make us live well, alert, mobile and independent, into our 80s.

Yet, what do we see? The majority of those over 60 are not mentally bright or physically fit and most are on medications, shuffling toward the Nursing Home.

In the third section of this Compendium or Book 3 "Successful Aging" you will see the incredible deterioration in our 'everyday' health such as our vision, hearing, lifting, walking, mobility, coping...unless you take preventive action now. Even if you are a teenager you should learn what to eat and to keep fit.

After discussing Premature Deaths, the major Premature Disabilities are then listed. These are preventable if we prevent or avoid premature deaths!

Successful Aging also lists the "minor" disabilities which can ruin our lives, and which are also mostly preventable.

FACTORS AFFECTING OUR HEALTH

Yes sure, we all know this! The only problem they are so familiar or obvious we disregard and discount them. Or we feel "it's our genes" – but our genes only account for some 6% to maybe 25% of our health issues.

So some 90% of living longer is up to you.

It would seem human nature that we prefer to take pills for our cholesterol, diabetes, blood pressure, depression and arthritis rather than achieving optimum weight which could cure all these – see Book 4 Slim 4 Life. Think about it!

a. **Established Health Criteria**
    1. Genetics
    2. Age
    3. Nutrition – the food we eat
    4. Weight
    5. Hygiene – mainly a clean water supply
    6. Environment – where we live – air pollution
    7. Medical markers – especially weight, blood pressure, lipids, blood and biochemical profile
    8. Exercise
    9. Mental status – personality, lack of stress, happiness, Alzheimer's
    10. Skin
    11. High-risk behaviours – as above
    12. Socio-economic-education status

b. **New Criteria: The "Missing Keys"**
    What and which illnesses and health problems occur *specific to age and sex or "What's Going to Kill You This Year"*.

The Missing Keys are those major conditions, peculiar to our age and sex, that cause our Premature Death or Disability or likely to kill you this year.

Heart attacks, Strokes, Depression, Diabetes, Arthritis and so on, all occur at different ages. If you know which and when, most can be avoided.
With respect to colon cancer): "Screening saves lives…90% are cured *if diagnosed and treated early enough."*
"Nine out of ten heart attacks can now be predicted."
"This suggests that approaches to prevention can be based on similar principles and have the potential to prevent most…."
"Life does not begin at 40" – but all serious illnesses do then take off like rockets and, again, by knowing this we can prevent them. And so on, for the majority of illnesses which cause our premature demise or disabilities.

Daily High Risk Behaviours that lead to early Illnesses, Injuries or Death

We now often just accept or don't recognize such behaviours as high risk. These are not the obvious testosterone-fueled risk taking by young men but are an insidious part of every-day modern life. However, they either shorten our lives or disable us.

This is not intended to wrap you in cotton wool but rather to alert you to pause and think how you may just improve here and there.

Processed Foods: We simply can't process Processed Foods. Since their introduction, after WW2, obesity and diabetes have become epidemics

Fat: You can call it obesity if you like but along with smoking and blood pressure it is the greatest cause of a reduced lifespan

Driving: road accidents take more lives than wars. Seat belts don't mean you can drive faster

Motorbikes: 5% of all vehicles, 25% of the accidents

Air Pollution: increasingly implicated in reduced lifespans

Sea Pollution: Microplastic ingestion ranges from 74,000 to 121,000 particles pa
        Fish increasingly contain higher levels of mercury

Waterways: Antibiotics, Antidepressants, cocaine etc are flushed into them

Environment: Pollution, traffic, factories, pesticides

Smoking: even second hand and even just one cigarette a day

Sun: Melanoma

Job: apart from the obvious outside workers e.g. carpenters, get more melanomas

Drinking: Increased incidence of many cancers as well as risky social behaviours

Sex: All STIs are on the increase and some resistant to all antibiotics

Contact sports: Footballers, boxers, higher rates of cognitive decline and Parkinsons Disease

Hygiene: Arguably at an all-time low as we think antibiotics will fix all – try Ebola, the flu

Travel: Malaria, food-poisoning

Medications: PPIs, Anticholinergics, Tranquillizers, Sleeping Tablets

Supplements & Vitamins: A proven waste of money unless obtained from foods.

SECTION D

CHAPTER 14.
WHO LIVES THE LONGEST

The Blue Zones:
Blue Zones was coined to identify a demographic or geographic area where people as a community (as distinct from individuals) live longer.

Five regions were identified

1. Sardinia, Italy (particularly Ogliastra, Barbagia di Ollolai and Barbagia of Seulo): one team of demographers found a hot spot of longevity in mountain villages where an amazing proportion of men reach the age of 100 years. In particular, a village located in the Barbagia of Seulo, holds the record of 20 centenarians from 1996 to 2016, that confirms it is " the place where people live the longest in the world "

2. Okinawa, Japan

3. Loma Linda, California: Seventh-day Adventists. But also Mormons.

4. Nicoya Peninsula, Costa Rica: A peninsula of long living men

5. Ikaria, Greece: has the highest percentage of 90-year-olds on the planet – nearly 1 out of 3 people make it to their 90s. Ikarians have about 20% lower rates of cancer, 50% lower rates of heart disease and almost no dementia.

6. Öland, Sweden - southern Småland and northeastern Skåne,

7. Acciaroli, Italy: one-third of its citizens (~ 300) live at least 80 years.

These people have in common a physical lifestyle, primitive plant-based diet and social integration.

People Who Live the Longest:
1. The Rich
2. Intelligence and Genetics
3. The Blue Zones
4. Adventists, Mormons
5. Individuals – see above
6. Nations – see above

Individual Longevity Top 100:

The USA: 50	Spain: 3
Japan: 19	Italy: 2
UK: 8	Australia:
France: 6	

What are the causes of disparities in longevity, and how can we live as long as the rich?

The examples of the Blue Zones of the world, where people, in general, live longest, would suggest that money is not the answer. Whereas, people, in general die early in the USA, individuals there, however, live longer, arguably because they are rich and can access the latest and best medical advice.

If the lifestyles of the Blue Zones and others who live longest are examined, they either have an enforced lifestyle such that they have to walk (no cars, hills), eat seasonal fresh foods (no refrigeration, no supermarkets), little meat, no processed foods because they are essentially isolated and poor or they have some religious imposts such as vegetarianism, no alcohol, no smoking or, if they are educated, they have adopted the essence of these healthier lifestyles.

While we can to a large extent mimic these conditions, the affluent West, with its processed foods, cars, and stressful long hours of work, has introduced new illnesses that cause premature deaths. In the West cardiovascular disease is our greatest killer, but it is relatively unknown in the Blue Zones, as are our next greatest killers, breast, prostate and colon cancer. Even if we try to mimic the Blue Zone ways with diet and exercise, our Western way of life is so pervasive that still we are struck down with unexpected "Western" illnesses, but the Adventists in California and the Mormons seem to be able to avoid them. But most of us who have no economic or religious imperatives imposed, will find it most difficult to adopt a default healthy lifestyle as our Western Society is geared to directly subvert and oppose it. This, of course, is not a sinister plot but simply the product of affluence and most of these illnesses that prematurely cause our demise or disabilities are, in fact, "Diseases of Affluence".

But now, in addition, and the point of this first Missing Keys book, is that, if we know what illnesses are most likely to strike us and when, then we can *also* take specific measures to avoid or minimize them.

This is Predictive Health Forecasting and allows for earlier Health Risk Identification and therefore better-focused, complete Prevention Plans for Successful Aging, Lifestyle, Nutrition, Exercise and Weight.

CHAPTER 15.
LIFE BEGINS AT 40?

Physical Declines Begin Earlier Than Expected

Physical declines begin sooner in life than when they become apparent, detected or obvious. Most often they are noticed when people are in their 40s, but the 'deterioration' has started much earlier.

Graphs (in the full Missing Keys book) dramatically show which and how most of these illnesses that prematurely kill or burden us, take off at the age of 40.

The conditions which 'suddenly' appear in middle age are:

1. Cardiovascular disease
2. Blood pressure
3. Cholesterol
4. Diabetes
5. Cancer
6. Lung disease
7. Rheumatoid arthritis
8. Osteoporosis / arthritis
9. Eyesight
10. Weight

While these major illnesses dramatically and suddenly make their appearance from age 40 they have been incubating but asymptomatic for many years. Damage may be in small doses, but it is cumulative... so it *"suddenly"* breaks out when we hit 40.

How can these be avoided?

Firstly, on the negative side, avoidance of High Risk Behaviours especially smoking, being sedentary and not eating processed foods. Secondly, on the positive side, eating good foods, being active, challenging yourself mentally and controlling your weight are fundamental. The aim is to maintain the ability to function independently. Physically, this can often be preserved with regular exercise. Efforts to maintain basic strength and endurance should begin before age 50, when it's still possible to preserve the skills that keep people mobile and independent later in life. In essence it is adopting, and most importantly, maintaining, a healthy lifestyle such that it becomes our norm.

SECTION E

DISABILITIES

CHAPTER 16.
PREMATURE DISABILITIES

"That which does not kill us, makes us stronger."
                                        Friedrich Nietzsche

However, what doesn't kill you, invariably makes you a premature invalid!

What Are Disabilities
Two aspects
    1. **Actual Practical Impediment**
    2. **Actual Medical Causative Conditions**

BOOK 3 Successful Aging has remarkable tables listing the progression of various Disabilities we are likely to encounter as we age. They are very salutary serving as warnings to avoid. Many are unvoiced: People are not likely to talk as to how they now find difficulty bathing but from age 18 years to 65 years it has become x 13 times more difficult! This was brought home to me when a 75year-old patient complained how he "could no longer wipe his bottom" - hardly something he is going to tell his friends but, more's the point, something he could have avoided had he known, as you can now, what Disabilities we are in for.

The Disabilities which show the greatest increases are: Hearing, walking three city Blocks, lifting 10 pounds (4.5kg), getting out of a chair, bathing, taking care of money, preparing meals or light housework.

Most, if not all of these can be avoided or considerably minimized.

If you know what Disabilities you are likely to encounter you can avoid, prevent or minimize them.

I am not talking minor stress. What I am talking about are major illnesses such as a stroke or a heart attack or an injury which, if the patient lives, condemns them to a greatly different, modified life, frequently dependent on others.

Both premature deaths and disabilities are obviously related...but they also differ.

One of the greatest causes of disabilities, which most of us don't even think about, is impaired hearing. These people may otherwise be in rude good health, but they are increasingly socially isolated and embarrassed. Deafness is a major disability.

Here there is a vast difference between death and disability.

Premature Death has been considered first but with the overlaps where death is avoided but disabilities result as with strokes. Disabilities are considered later and in greater detail in the third book of this Compendium.

> *Over 1 in 4 of today's 20year-olds will become disabled before they retire*

USA
Over 37 million Americans are classified disabled; ~ 12% of the total population.
More than 50% are in their working years, from 18-64.

UK
There are 12.9 million disabled people in the UK.
7 per cent of children are disabled
17 per cent of working age adults are disabled
45 per cent of pension age adults are disabled
The most commonly reported impairments by disabled people are:
  1. Mobility (53%)
  2. Stamina, breathing, fatigue (39%)
  3. Dexterity (29%).

AUSTRALIA
In Australia 18.5% reported having a disability in 2009, according to the results of the Survey of Disability, Ageing and Carers (SDAC). For the purposes of SDAC, disability is defined as any limitation, restriction or impairment which restricts everyday activities and has lasted or is likely to last for at least six months. Examples range from loss of sight that is not corrected by glasses, to arthritis which causes difficulty dressing, to advanced dementia that requires constant help and supervision. Males and females were similarly affected by disability (18% and 19% respectively)

Disabilities
The Center for Disease Control estimates some 20% of the population in the United States (but applicable to all first world countries) is living with a disability and increases as new disability categories such as neurodiversity, psychiatric disabilities, disabilities of aging and learning disabilities emerge. The three most common causes of disability in the USA continued to be arthritis or rheumatism, back or spine problems and heart trouble. Women (24.4%) had a significantly higher prevalence of disability compared with men (19.1%) at all ages. For both sexes, the prevalence of disability doubled in successive age groups (18--44 years, 11.0%; 45--64 years, 23.9%; and ≥65 years, 51.8%)

CHAPTER 17.
MALE AND FEMALE: OVERALL

When young high risk and even low risk (but cumulative) behaviors are often treated as a "rite of passage' or relegated to be addressed when older. Drinking and now binge drinking are epidemic. Smoking has gratifyingly been recognized as 'not cool' but a stupid, injurious affectation and drug of addiction.

Cars pull up beside me with speakers that would do Carnegie Hall justice with some young man with a baseball cap on backwards gyrating to the beat, which seems to lift his car off the ground but ensuring his accelerated hearing loss. Meanwhile in my rear-vision mirror some 18year-old or so girl is tailgating me until she cuts me off with the one-finger salute and absolutely no idea how to control a skid. And both of these are drinking a Cola and eating pizza or some processed food and are overweight. The only exercise they get is their thumbs texting on their Smart-Phones. They have little or no idea of nutrition or hygiene and getting a tan is most desirable.

While Sir William Osler observed how humans have a great desire to take pills, as a doctor there is simply no-way I could ever take something made by some criminal without any quality control or guaranteed dose. That is simply crazy - suicidal in fact.

I have no answer to these behaviours other than alerting those readers under 40 years of age, or their parents or anyone (!) to these avoidable disorders let alone fatal illnesses.

Of course, I was perfect and never indulged in such practices...Pig's Bottom...I often say the only reason I'm alive is that when I arrived at the Pearly Gates (or was it the other place) the "Use-By-Date" on my forehead was blurred and they sent me back.

But a friend of mine, a Rock 'N Roll Drummer, who, of course has a hearing loss, told me how he "wished someone had told him to wear ear-plugs and the dangers of loud noise". But I don't think he would have listened - (bad pun).

But hopefully a word in a not yet hearing-impaired ear at least may alert and prevent this avoidable damage.

The Earlier You Start, the Less Downstream Problems

Premature Deaths and Disabilities

Tobacco – cigarette smoking

Processed foods

Eating habits – processed and junk foods – lack of fruit/vegetables

Exercise patterns – physical inactivity

High blood pressure

Drinking habits – alcohol harm

Weight – overweight/underweight

High LDL

Driving style

Hobbies – high risk - head trauma from sport

Occupations – high risk

Pesticides, industrial-workplace toxins (nail salons)

Diesel fumes / Air pollution

Unsafe sex

Illicit drugs

Lack of vaccinations

Hygiene

Loud music, noise

Glare

Sunburn

CHAPTER 18.
WHAT'S UP, DOC?

Prevalent Health Problems: Why We Go to The Doctor (%)

1. Dental caries --
2. Hearing loss 16
3. Endentulism (loss of teeth) 7.6
4. Asthma 6.6
5. Periodontal D 5.6
6. Iron anemia 4
7. Alcohol abuse 4
8. Osteoarthritis 3
9. Chronic Back pain 3.2
10. Depression 3
11. Diabetes 2 2.6
12. Slipped disc 1.9
13. Incontinent urine 1.7
14. Chronic Obstructive Pulmonary Disease (COPD) 1.6
15. Social phobia 1.6
16. Anxiety disorder 1.6
17. Burns/scalds 1.3
18. Benign Prostatic Hypertrophy 1.1
19. Peptic ulcer 1.0
20. Attention Deficit D (ADD) 0.9
21. Cannabis abuse 0.9
22. Cataracts 0.9
23. Angina 0.9
24. Osteoporosis 0.8
25. Bipolar Disorder 0.7

Reasons for Attending the Doctor per 1000 patients

URTIs 2370 (Upper Respiratory Tract Infections)
Dental Caries 594
Chronic. Back pain 330
Diarrhea 205
LRTIs 190 (Lower Respiratory Tract Infections)
Otitis media 56
Periodontal Disease 22
Depression 21
Falls 20
Skin cancers 15
Alcohol abuse 9
Peptic ulcer 9
Slipped disc 8
Hearing loss 6
Menstrual problems 6
Motor Vehicle Accident (MVA) 5
Diverticulitis 4
Anxiety disorder 4
Sports injuries 4
Asthma 4
Gall bladder Disease 4
Stroke 3
Prostate hypertrophy 3
Interpersonal violence 3
Angina

Reasons Attending the Doctor (%) one decade later

Check-up 9
Prescription 7.1
Cough 4.5
Test results 3.6
Vaccination 3.1
Sore throat 2.5
Back complaint 2.3
Rash 1.9
Fever 1.5
URTI 1.4

Headache 1.4
Abdominal pain 1.3
Depression 1.3
Hypertension 1.2
Nasal problem 1.2
Ear pain 1.1
Diarrhea 1.0
Tiredness 1.0
Administrative 1.0
Knee complaint 0.9

Most Managed Problems by the Doctor (%)

Hypertension 6.1
URTI 4.4
Vaccination 3.2
Depression 2.4
Lipid disorder 2.1
Diabetes 2.0
Back pain 1.8
Bronchitis 1.8
Osteoarthritis 1.8

Prescription 1.4
Check-up 1.3
Esophageal Disease 1.3
Female genital/pap 1.2
Sprain 1.2
Urinary Tract Infection 1.2
Sleep problems 1.1
Anxiety 1.1
Menopausal symptoms 1

Most Commonly Reported Long-Term Conditions aka "Disabilities"

CONDITION	MALE %	FEMALE %	TOTAL %
Long-sightedness	20.4	24.3	22.4
Short-sightedness	18.3	23.5	20.9
Back pain / disc disorders	21.0	20.7	20.9
Hay fever / allergic rhinitis	15.1	15.9	15.6
Arthritis (all forms)	11.7	15.8	13.9
Asthma	10.5	12.6	11.6
Chronic sinusitis	8.9	12.4	10.5
Deafness (total/partial)	14.2	7.7	10.8
Hypertension	9.7	10.7	10.3
Presbyopia	9.1	9.0	9.0
Migraine	3.6	8.7	6.2
High cholesterol	6.5	5.6	6.1
Astigmatism	3.9	5.3	4.6
Anxiety disorders	3.4	5.6	4.5
Mood disorders	3.4	5.5	4.5
Bronchitis/emphysema	3.5	3.6	3.6
Diabetes (all forms)	3.0	2.9	3.0
GIT ulcers	2.8	2.7	2.7
Varicose veins	1.1	3.5	2.3
Hernia	2.5	1.6	2.0
Cataract	1.5	2.4	2.0
Tachycardia	1.7	2.1	1.9
Psoriasis	1.5	2.0	1.8
Neoplasms/cancers	2.0	1.4	1.7
Osteoporosis	0.6	2.5	1.6
Edema	1.0	2.1	1.6
Angina	1.6	1.2	1.4
Rheumatism	1.3	1.4	1.3
Anemias	0.3	2.3	1.3
Hemorrhoids	1.0	1.2	1.1
Dermatitis/eczema	1.0	1.2	1.1

SECTION F

CHAPTER 19.
EARLY DIAGNOSIS & TREATMENT

> Get It Seen, Get It Diagnosed, Get It Fixed

History & Examination
The difference between the *Live Longest* check-up and an ordinary annual check-up is that it focuses on those illnesses most likely to affect you and takes into account the age group of the patient.

Some investigation require specialized equipment—eye, mammograms Examinations of the following systems are recommended.

Preliminary Measurements:
Height and weight, BMI, Waist
Skin – dermoscopy – regular checks in Sunbelt areas
Cardiovascular
Central nervous system
Respiratory system
Gastro intestinal system
Genito-urinary System: male/female
Endocrine
ENT (Ear, Nose, Throat). Eyes – visual acuity and fields, fundi.
Hearing – auditory acuity
Musculoskeletal/Locomotor
Psychiatric/Mental
Age grip, mobility, posture, nutrition, hydration, feet, walk speed

Medical Symptoms & Signs
The earlier an illness can be diagnosed the more chance of a cure. It is therefore important for you to know what symptoms and signs to look for and not to ignore them. The following is a list of the main signs and symptoms which to report.

General
Undue fatigue or tiredness
Unexplained loss of weight
Unexplained bruising / prolonged bleeding
Any blood transfusions
Slowness of movement or mental process
Eyes
Grittiness / inflammation / watering / discharge
Pain & blurring
Loss of vision. Stuck lids
Recent overseas travel

GIT (Gastro Intestinal Tract)

Heartburn/indigestion	Weight loss
Abdominal pain	Yellow whites of eyes
Change of bowel habit	Recurrent diarrhoea
PR mucus, blood, slime	Intolerance to bread

CVS (Cardiovascular System)

Blood pressure	Chest pain
Palpitations/fluttering	Swollen ankles
SOBOE (Shortness of breath on effort)	

Respiratory

Smoking	Bad snoring / choking in sleep
Persistent cough / blood in sputum	Any previous exposure to asbestos
Wheeze / asthma / difficulty breathing	

CNS (Central Nervous System)

KOd	Disturbances of balance
Transient loss of vision / consciousness	New headache
(TIA)	Tremors
Altered behavior	Increasing forgetfulness / confusion
Fits	Progressivly smaller writing
Pins and needles	Reduced sense of smell
Weakness of grip	

Locomotor / Muscle or joints

Pain	Increasing tendency to choke on food
Swelling	Unaccounted for limp
Inflammation	Finger nodes
Joint pains – note any climbing stairs	Weaker grip

Endocrine

Slowing down (compared with 1 year ago)
Thinning hair
Menstrual problems
Pop eyes
Fast talk
Central obesity
Thirst, polyuri

Men

Diminished stream & cut off
Frequency/nocturia
Terminal dribbling
Pink urine
Testicular lumps
Early erection difficulties

Work

Exposure to asbestos, diesel, pesticides, sun

Women

Any lump
Mammogram/pap
Stress incontinence
Frequency/nocturia
Cystitis/pink urine
Discharge / Inter-menstrual bleeding

Age

Trouble getting out of chairs
Increasingly fixed opinions
Memory problems
Feet – not cared for
Back pain

Mental Health

Feeling something is wrong
Sadness / hopelessness / worthlessness
Worried all the time
Loss of interest
Inappropriate guilt
Sleep difficulties
Suicidal thoughts
Memory problems
Repetition

CHAPTER 20.
TESTS & INVESTIGATIONS

Medical tests and investigations are important tools in the early diagnosis of potentially life-threatening and/or debilitating illnesses. It is the *Live Longest* contention that screening tests must be specific tests focused for your age and sex.

In 2001, the Director of the Center for Disease Control in Atlanta, USA (the NASA of medicine) declared (with respect to colon cancer): "Screening saves lives... 90% are cured if diagnosed and treated early enough."

"Nine out of ten heart attacks can now be predicted."

"This finding suggests that approaches to prevention can be based on similar principles and have the potential to prevent most premature cases of myocardial infarction."

The challenge is to select those tests that are cost-effective. They should give an answer as to where a cure or improvement can be made, given your age. It is important that both the patient and physician realize the necessity, desirability and usefulness of all investigations and any risks involved (such as with CT scans).

What Tests Should Be Done
There is a battery of tests appropriate for each age group and sex. "Common things occur most commonly"—so it is most important (at least six times as important) to screen your cardiac risks. Rare or expensive tests should only be done if your history and examination suggests they are necessary or if you wish to pay for it to satisfy your curiosity or anxiety. The basic tests that follow do not carry any significant risks. If you do need further complex tests, then any risks should be fully explained.

ECG/EKGs and stress testing have long been considered by many cardiologists as part of CVS screening. But are they predictive and cost-effective? Probably not. Would you have them done? Probably yes.
Some screening tests such as mammography and pap smears have been introduced as "recommended" but debate has raged as to cost-effectiveness and restrictions have been invariably imposed to attract a rebate.
Meanwhile a FBC (Full Blood Count) and MBA (Multiple Biochemical Analysis) are so ubiquitous that they are accepted as "necessary" when often they are not.

Medicine often gets caught trying to be all things to all people. However, the following tests and investigations are considered to be both cost-effective and evidenced. These should be undertaken on the judgement of the clinician. Any abnormalities progress to secondary tests.

Recommended Age-Specific Tests Selected From:
- Blood and biochemical FBC/ESR/CRP, MBA including Blood Glucose
- Cardiovascular check – Cholesterol HDL:LDL, Triglycerides, ECG/EKG annually over 65
- Prostate check
- Gynecology check – Pap, Mammogram, DEXA
- Colon cancer check – Colonoscopy (age 50 or 40 if smoking, drinking, male)
- Skin check – dermoscopy
- Coeliac D – IgA TTG and serum IgA
- Metabolic and others – as indicated from history and examination
- Chest x-ray (PA & lateral)

What These Tests Are and What They Are For

1. Hematology: FBC = Full Blood Count
- Hemoglobin – indicates if you are anemic
- White Cell Count – indicates infection, leukemia
- ESR – indicates inflammation
- Platelet Count – indicates bleeding problems
- CRP – indicates inflammation

2. Biochemistry: MBA = Multiple Biochemical Analysis
- Sodium, potassium, chloride, bicarbonate, anion gap, osmolality are the electrolytes which compose the body fluids & their balance
- Calcium/Phosphate/Alkaline phosphatase – bone disorders
- Urea & Creatinine – indicate kidney function
- Urate – elevated in gout & metabolic syndrome in children & adolescents
- Glucose – elevated in Diabetes
- Protein (Albumin and Globulin) – low in kidney and some liver disease and high in some metabolic disorders (Myeloma)
- Bilirubin – indicates gall bladder/liver disease
- The "ase(s)" are enzymes which indicate liver and sometimes heart problems
- Iron – low in blood loss – from piles to cancer

3. Lipids

Cholesterol – good HDL and bad LDL. Elevated LDL(microglobules) considered a major heart risk

Triglycerides – one of the lipids – elevation considered a heart risk

4. *Coeliac Disease Antibodies* – see section on Coeliac Disease, sequel book.

5. Colonoscopy/Endoscopy

A camera on the end of a photo-optic cable is inserted via the anus to examine the lower gut. Patients are mostly sedated and the actual procedure is painless. It can detect Cancer of the Colon (CAC) early enough to effect a cure. FOBT (Fecal Occult Blood Tests) are blotting paper tests on your feces for minute amounts of blood. They are cheaper, less embarrassing but not as good. Colonoscopy is "The Gold Standard."
Endoscopes are passed via the mouth into the stomach to look for ulcers or cancers.

6. *Other specific tests as indicated* (e.g., Thyroid Function)

7. *ECG/EKG:* Detects any abnormalities of heart rhythm and rate at rest and evidence of any old infarcts.

8. Cardiac Stress Test

This determines any sinister changes with exercise and if okay, indicates that exercise does not provoke dangerous changes.

9. Coronary Scoring

Detects any calcium in coronary arteries, which is one indicator of degenerative disease. It is of some 51% help with respect to predicting acute cardiac events (heart attacks); that is, it is not the full answer. However, it further helps provide more information about the most important aspect of our health (our heart). It has now been found to be helpful even in those younger than 50 years

10. *PSA* – Prostate-Specific Antigen

Indicates either prostate enlargement—Benign Prostatic Enlargement (BPH)—or cancer.

PSA presents an ethical problem in that, if it is elevated, it is not diagnostic; so you are then faced with the dilemma, according to your age, as to what to do. You can investigate further and if it is cancer, have treatment which often leads to impotence and incontinence; or, let it go, as it is very slow growing, and the average duration of life if untreated is another 10 years. Thus if you are 50 you have a decision; but if you are 70 maybe not. According to the above philosophy, if you get it done, you may choose to repeat it every 5 years or so. The one laboratory keeps a comparative record which is preferable to having it done elsewhere.

11. DEXA: This is a special x-ray to detect osteoporosis. Heel-bone densities are not satisfactory.

12. Dermoscopy
These are hand-held or cable-optic cameras that optically take away the top layer of skin so the examiner can see better the histology of the mole or skin lesion underneath; it enhances the diagnosis of melanoma and skin cancers.

Normal Values
The United States reports many values in mg/liter, where the United Kingdom, Europe, Australia and New Zealand use mom/l. All laboratories give their normal range after the test specimen results. Normal values may differ between labs.

This table of tests is only a guide and represents screening at a first attendance.

Some tests may not need to be repeated. After a baseline around 20 years, lipids should be done every 5 years. 10-year screening otherwise is suggested, reducing to 5-year intervals after 45 years or as clinically assessed.

Age Specific Tests

AGE	MALE	FEMALE
15-30	CXR (PA & lateral) FBC/ESR/CRP, MBA Coeliac D Cardiovascular check Others as indicated STD (4% asymptomatic)	CXR (PA & lateral) FBC/ESR/CRP, MBA Coeliac D Cardiovascular check Gynecology (Pap, breasts, STD) Others as indicated
30-40	CXR (PA & lateral) FBC/ESR/CRP, MBA Coeliac D Cardiovascular check incl. LDL Others as indicated	CXR (PA & lateral) FBC/ESR/CRP, MBA Coeliac D Cardiovascular check incl. LDL Gynecology Pap smear, breasts Others as indicated
40-50	CXR (PA & lateral) FBC/ESR/CRP, MBA Coeliac D Cardiovascular check Prostrate check Colon Cancer Others as indicated Coronary Scoring	CXR (PA & lateral) FBC/ESR/CRP, MBA Coeliac D Cardiovascular check Gynecology (Pap, mammogram, DEXA) Colon Cancer Others as indicated Coronary Scoring
50–64	CXR (PA & lateral) FBC/ESR/CRP, MBA Coeliac D Cardiovascular check Prostrate check Colon Cancer Others as indicated Hearing Coronary Scoring	CXR (PA & lateral) FBC/ESR/CRP, MBA Coeliac D Cardiovascular check Gynecology Colon Cancer Others as indicated Vision Coronary Scoring
65–74	ECG/EKG annual – exclude AF Ultrasonography for Abdominal Aortic Aneurysm Coronary Scoring	ECG/EKG annually – exclude AF Coronary Scoring

ADDENDA

Drugs: I have so many nice, well balanced, hard-working patients in my practice who, much to my surprise, contracted Hepatitis C, which means they were injecting illicit drugs when young. They are all embarrassed and sheepish about it now but, thank goodness, Hep C is now curable. And while they all claim they regret it, and wouldn't do it again, the temptation must have been so great that even these ostensibly well-adjusted people were tempted to try drugs.
Just don't. They all have long term damage.

Tattoos: Tatts are as old as the world and usually of tribal symbolic culture. Fashion goes in vogues and today, most young people are encouraged to join the crowd and get a Tat …and then another.
However, to my experience my patients, both male and female, express a universal regret when they reach middle or old age and what may have seemed exciting and fashionable in one's 20s is now rather embarrassing and pathetic in one's 50s. Many then spend a small fortune trying to have them removed.
Resist the temptation and see if you still want one when you are 50.

Tans
Tanned skin was a marker of the outdoor worker and peasants, but the Industrial Revolution saw these workers now pushed indoors into factories and, in the 1920s, Coco Chanel made us admire and desire a tan as only the rich could then afford luxury holidays in the south of France.
Melanoma then became 'the only disease the rich got more than the poor'.
There is no such thing as a 'safe' tan.

Suicide and accidental poisoning leading cause of death for 20-34 year olds
Suicide (including injury/poisoning of undetermined intent) was the leading cause of death for 20 - 34 year olds (24% of men and 12% of women). Factors that could lead to these deaths include: Traumatic experiences, lifestyle choices such as drug or alcohol misuse, job insecurity and relationship problems. For both sexes, accidental poisoning is also a highly common cause of death, followed by land transport accidents.

Breast cancer leading cause of death for 35 - 49 year old women
Breast cancer is the leading cause of death among women in this age group, accounting for 14% of deaths. However, it is the leading cause because women in this age group are relatively healthy and are therefore less likely to die of other causes. Breast cancer deaths in women aged 15-49 years only account for around 10% of all female breast cancer deaths.

Suicide remains the leading cause of death for men aged 35-49, accounting for 13% of deaths.

Heart disease leading cause of death for men aged 50 and over

For those aged 50 and over, the leading causes of death for both men and women were long-term diseases and conditions. Cancer of the trachea, bronchus and lung is the number one cause for women aged 50-64, accounting for 11% of deaths in this group. Breast cancer is the 2nd leading cause of death for 50-64year old women, accounting for 11% of deaths in this age group. Heart diseases are the leading cause of death for men aged 50 and over. Lifestyle choices and other conditions can lead to heart disease such as: smoking, high cholesterol, high blood pressure and diabetes.

Dementia and Alzheimer's leading cause of death for women over 80

Dementia and Alzheimer's disease was the leading cause of death for women over 80 accounting for 17% of deaths and was the second leading cause for men causing 11% of deaths in this age group. Deaths from dementia and Alzheimer's disease are increasing as people live longer and are more common in women as women live longer than men. The leading cause of death for men in this age group was ischaemic heart disease accounting for 15% of deaths, this was the second leading cause for women causing 11% of deaths In the UK around 6% of children are disabled, compared to 16% of working age adults and 45% of adults over State Pension age.

Two Decade Analysis Reveals Risk Factors Are on the Rise Despite Greater Awareness

Despite increased understanding of heart disease risk factors and the need for preventive lifestyle changes, patients suffering the most severe type of heart attack (ST-elevation myocardial infarction, or STEMI) have become younger, more obese and more likely to have preventable risk factors such as smoking, high blood pressure, diabetes and chronic obstructive pulmonary disease.

Whereas in 1999, cardiovascular disease (CVD) excluding stroke was the main cause of death in all US states except Alaska, 14 years later, deaths from cancer surpassed those from CVD in almost half of the states, a new study reports.

About half of the dramatic reduction in heart-disease mortality can be attributed to better treatments such as revascularization, and about half to reductions in risk factors such as smoking, cholesterol, and blood pressure, but not BMI or diabetes.

BOOK 4

SLIM 4 LIFE

Even the Svelte Benefit from Eating Less

In adults already at a healthy weight or carrying just a few extra pounds, cutting around 300 calories a day significantly improved already good levels of cholesterol, blood pressure, blood sugar and other markers. *The Lancet Diabetes & Endocrinology July 11, 2019.*

MEASUREMENTS

We will use calories as the unit (not kilojoules)

Scales, a tape measure and a mirror are all you need

Aim: to get a flat tummy

SUCCESS

**91% success rate is possible for Long Term weight loss
Long Term is 30 kg over 10 years**

The DANGEROUS VISCERAL FAT

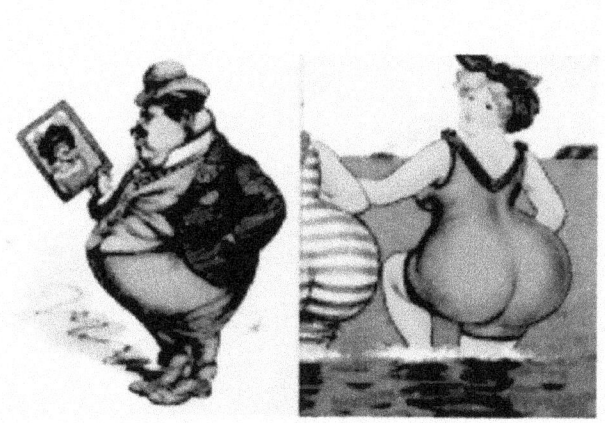

Apple and Pear

The dangerous fat is the Visceral Fat which is deep and surrounds our organs. Men are apple shaped which has the more metabolically harmful (waist) Visceral Fat.

Women are Pear shaped which is metabolically protective (hips) but worse than for men if they gain waist fat. However, making obesity an object of humor has impeded understanding the medical consequences. It has been found essential for health, no matter your height, to have:

Waist circumference: Women < 90 cm
                                  Men   < 102 cm

- Obesity has almost tripled worldwide since 1975,
- Obese people outnumber smokers by 2:1 and overtakes smoking as the leading cause of cancer
- BMI has increased for both genetically predisposed and non-predisposed people, implying that the environment remains the main contributor
- Most of us eat more when we exercise, and though it may be just a few extra bites a day, the result is weight gain.

SLIM 4 LIFE COMPENDIUM GUIDE

BED: Behavior, Exercise, Diet -Nutrition

A. **RECOMMENDED DIETS (select one to suit)**
   1. Reduce all meals every day (ED) by a minimum 10% up to 25%.
   2. Do Intermittent Fasting (IF) (500 - 600 calories) two days a week
   3. 16:8 Eat for 8 hours fast for 16 hours (no breakfast)

B. **BEHAVIOUR-LIFESTYLE**
   COMMIT: Determination, Dedication, Discipline, Resolve, Restraint

C. **MOTIVATION**
   Mindful Eating
   Stay Motivated
   How to Keep Dieting

D. **MAINTENANCE**
   Monitoring
   Traps
   Disillusionment
   Not Losing

E. **HINTS, TRICKS AND GOOD ADVICE**

F. **BENEFITS**

NEWTRITION Book 2

EXERCISE Book 5

WHY ARE WE SO FAT?

We are the fattest generation in the history of the world.

Why?

This obesity epidemic only started in the 1980s and our genes haven't changed, nor has our microbiome.

What then has changed?

Our food has altered more in the past 65 years than the previous 650,000 and it is delicious, cheap and available 24 hours a day, seven days a week, 365 days a year. Whereas Food used to be scarce, meat rationed, famines often.

The need for 'compressed' rations for the soldiers in WW2 heralded the development of processed foods and synthetic additives, and now over 85,000 new chemicals have been introduced with over 87,000 "health" supplements on the market today.

Many, if not most, of these are untested and, whereas we humans slowly evolved to know what we needed to eat (and what not to eat) and which took millions of years, these processed foods have all been developed, only in the last 65 years. I feel we humans simply have not had time to adapt to them. My hypothesis would now seem to be being supported as recent studies are now finding that these processed foods reduce lifespan and contribute to heart disease. It has been my contention, long before this research, that we simply "can't process, processed foods" and that this affects our whole metabolic cycles, not only our heart, and that they insidiously put on fat and cause other metabolic disorders such as Diabetes 2.

We now live in a toxic-obesogenic society with this processed food costing three times less than fresh food and available 24 hours a day, seven days a week, home delivered, unrelentingly advertised, and tastes delicious.

Americans are eating 736 more calories a day than previous generations but now the whole civilized world is eating 650 calories more, every day. But we only need 20 more calories a day to gain weight and 100 a day to become obese.

And we don't have to walk, run, dig, lift, chop or do anything as physical as our Grandparents or Parents. We are also the most sedentary generation in history.

The researched reasons why people want to lose weight list "To look good" as number one with "Health" down at number four. However, a recent trial in the UK found that people who had Diabetes 2 (T2D) *did* make health number one because they were so sick and tired of taking tablets.

We now suffer the Diseases of Affluence: Obesity, High Blood Pressure (Hypertension), Heart Attacks, Strokes, Diabetes 2, Hyperlipidaemia (cholesterol), Arthritis, Depression and many more. Most, however, can be improved by losing just 10% of weight and many cured.

Losing weight long term is possible. In fact, a 81% success rate is possible.

Long-term is defined as a loss of 30lb for over a year.

There is no one diet that works for everyone. Dieting, for most, means restrictive selection of foods. Diets have been recorded and duplicated for over 2,500 years. They are duplicated or repeated every so often as the "new" fad. They all work – short term, however, to lose weight long-term more than just food selection is needed. A whole system is needed.

S4L provides this unique 4 System Total Weight Loss Program comprising 4 elements
  1. Diet
  2. Behaviour
  3. Nutrition
  4. Exercise

The acronym for this is BED (Behaviour, Exercise, Diet) + Nutrition

You will have to find the diet that suits you and you can stick to. This requires some experimenting and S4L makes recommendations which are best.

So the first steps are
  1. Find an eating program (a diet) that you can stick to
  2. Learn what healthy foods are
  3. Don't eat any processed – junk foods

The hardest part, however is
  4. Behaviour modification
  5. Exercise is most important but it only accounts for some 15%

Losing weight is arguably the hardest thing to do but, what is also hard, is trying to condense all the detail of my whole book into this summary – so I urge you to get the whole book – and to keep reading and reading it to keep motivated.

HOW DO WE GET FAT

Do you inhale fat cells? Or, when you are asleep, do the Fat Elves slip under the gap under your door and inject cellulite? Or what?

While it is now medically 'fashionable' to blame our genes and gut microbiome, they have not changed, yet we are witnessing a new epidemic of Obesity. This was only first noticed in the 1980s, some 20 years after WW2 and following the invention spurt and mass marketing of processed foods.

Only the food, and amount we eat has changed, not our genes or gut flora.

That said, genes do play a part in some 6% of the population.

This is not a book for the medically obese, nor for this 6%, but for those of us who were once slim but have now insidiously put on weight and are having difficulties taking it off.

Maybe that's 94% of us!
    Weight = Food intake minus exercise
    Excess Food = Fat Excess

or, more accurately,
    Fat = Food Type (Processed Junk) minus exercise

And exercise doesn't lose much (but is essential).
    Food   = 85%
    Exercise = 15%

We cannot create fat out of thin air, we can only convert it from food.

If we eat more than our metabolic needs, food then converts into fat.

There are many, many contributors to us gaining weight, some are more prone than others, and obesity is a profound medical problem. But for most of us we are simply overeating and eating the wrong (processed) foods. And, what I do not want is for anyone blaming their genes, their microbiome, their parents, their stress or anything else as the cause of their being overweight when they are eating more than they can metabolise.

I am not being cruel or unsympathetic here. Losing weight is arguably the hardest thing we can attempt, and we need massive support but also insight that we are overeating. However, we may not realise it, may not even know we are doing it. Most of us have been insidiously just eating 20 calories a day more but we can eat 1,000 cals more and not realise it! We don't know how to identify any excess let alone make adjustments and don't know how to make the essential changes to our lifestyle and not just blindly follow a fad diet.

To that end S4L provides a whole support program and not just a diet.

If you blame your propensity for being lardy on your genes, the latest scientific findings may come as a blow. At last month's (May 2019) American Society for Nutrition conference in Baltimore researchers revealed that while we can hold our parents responsible for many things in life, piling on the kilograms isn't likely to be one of them.

In the Predict study results showed that body responses to different foods, measured by levels of glucose, fats and hormones in the blood, were widely different, even for the identical twins. No two people processed fats and carbohydrates in the same way and less than half of the variation in their biochemical reaction to the food could be attributed to genetic influences.

Only about 30 per cent of the glucose response that occurs after a meal was genetic according to our latest estimate and virtually zero, or at least less than 5 per cent, for fat.

It explains why some people will lose weight on one diet while others won't and why I recommend you now keep trying the diet that works best for you.

Experiment with the timing and composition of your meals and with time-restricted eating where you have a specified eating window each day.

CHAPTER 1.
RECOMMENDED DIETS

1. Reduce all meals by 10% (min) to 25% (leave 1/3 of the food on your plate). A stricter version is only 800 cals a day which achieves faster results.
2. Intermittent Fasting (500 to 600 cals) two non-sequential days a week
3. 16:8 No eating after 8pm until 12 noon

There are minor variations to these.

45% of successful long-term dieters used their own.
Most tried several diets before they found the one that suited them.

Most other diets are fads and scams.

PERSONALISED DIETS

As in the PREDICT Study People react differently to same food eg Blood Glucose (BG) response
This has led to commercial enterprises offering "Personalised Diets" but while there may be something to it, it is too early and such proposed diets are dubious.
You may wish, however, to buy a Glucometer and measure your own levels.

EXPECTATIONS

Have real expectations. Initially just aim for 1kg at a time.
Long-term try to lose 5%.
Then reassess.

300 Calories Less per day – even if you are healthy
Reducing daily food intake by the equivalent of just a couple of cookies, or around 300 calories, over 2 years leads to improvements in body composition and a range of cardiometabolic risk factors that would result in reductions in the incidence of cardiovascular disease

NOT RECOMMENDED

Keto Diet (see complete book):
Anti-social, too hard to maintain, better alternatives and a repeated fad started in 1911 (again see complete book)

Paleo Diet
Many Paleo diet proponents claim the diet is beneficial to gut health, but recent research suggests that when it comes to the production of TMAO in the gut, an organic compound produced in the gut, which is associated with an increased risk of heart disease, the Paleo diet could be having an adverse impact in terms of heart health. The Paleo diet includes greater servings per day of red meat, which provides the precursor compounds to produce TMAO, and Paleo followers consumed twice the recommended level of saturated fats, which is cause for concern. In addition, the Paleo diet excludes all grains and whole grains are a fantastic source of resistant starch and many other fermentable fibres that are vital to the health of the gut microbiome, and because TMAO is produced in the gut, a lack of whole grains might change the populations of bacteria enough to enable higher production of this compound. *European Journal of Nutrition 2019.*

CHAPTER 2.
BEHAVIOUR MODIFICATION

This is the hardest of the four elements in the Slim 4 Life program.

Commitment: Think this through.

You don't stand a chance unless you can selfishly devote your whole lifestyle to this. You will need determination, dedication, discipline, resolve and restraint.

If you have a hectic social life, birthdays coming up, stress from work, financial problems, family issues, illness, holidays, a partner who can't or won't help or anything that can sabotage your eating less, forget it OR make 'secret' plans to avoid these traps.

This IS possible: There are many, many lean people who are stressed, bad sleepers, love sweet junk foods, have high pressure jobs and are asked to parties, business lunches and dinners every week. But they have a plan and don't just pig out or be tempted "just this time".

So, think ahead. What commitments are coming up and how will (not 'can') you eat and drink less at these events.

Remember, everyone wants to tempt you off your diet so don't tell them. When they plonk a huge meal in front of you make sure you leave a 1/3 and have an excuse such as 'That was fantastic- I'm so sorry I had that big lunch which was nowhere as nice but I now can't eat another thing" ...or some such.

Finally, while it may sound silly, if you are determined not to eat say until 6pm (a fixed objective time), you will not feel hungry; but if you constantly brood, think of food and are bored you are entering a self-defeating spiral.

But if you are not committed, don't think ahead and not determined to stick to your plan, you are doomed to stay as you are or even put on more weight as you won't face the fact that you are eating too much because you give in to temptation.

"I can resist anything except temptation" - Oscar Wilde.

The key is to identify the habits, temptations, routines, triggers and traps that stimulate you to eat and make it easier for you to do so.

The classic is where we get home from work and go to the fridge, get a snack and have a drink. But there are many, many more triggers that get us to eat.

Think as to your present behavior and then how you can alter the food-eating aspects as in

- Don't have any snacks after 8pm
- Small controlled snacks only to abate hunger / cravings
- Don't have any food in the house. Essentials only
- No processed foods whatsoever – ever!
- Alter your routine(s). Do Something Different (DSD)
- Eat much more slowly

CHAPTER 3.
MOTIVATION

Researched Motivations
1. Appearance. To look better; have more sex appeal
2. To improve self-esteem, pride, confidence
3. To feel better, have more energy
4. To be healthier and live longer
5. To have more control over one's life
6. To fit into smaller clothes
7. Personal goals – an anniversary, marriage
8. Overheard criticism
9. To get less discrimination; more pay
10. For a bet

Get Motivated
Motivation to lose weight may best be defined, as "giving a person the reason, enthusiasm and determination, to change weight gaining to weight losing, behavior(s)".
Being motivated is arguably the most important key to losing weight. The Reasons why we want to lose weight are listed below but these are not quite the same as being motivated.

Why We Overeat
This is one step before the listed Motivators.
- What feelings cause you to eat
    - Hunger
    - Stress
    - Depression
    - Addiction – Binge eating
    - Boredom
- Others
    - Habits
    - Availability of food especially in house
    - Medications
- Re-set of previous normal intake
    - Chronic insidious little bit more each day
    - Processed foods
    - Obesogenic environment

Analyzing and thinking about these will help you address these stimuli.

MINDFUL EATING

Mindfulness has been defined as the act of focusing attention on present moment experiences. With respect to eating it means concentrating and paying attention to the food you are eating as opposed to 'just shoveling it in' with your mind and conversation elsewhere.

The object is to think about every mouthful or food you are putting in your mouth rather than being distracted or thinking of something else, some problem, work, TV, the phone or whatever. Think more about fullness cues and leaving food.

12 Recommendations

1. Make eating an exclusive event. When you eat – only eat. Give eating the attention it needs to fully enjoy your food and be mindful of every bite. Without distraction you better recognize when you are full.
2. Check your stress level. Eating is a common response to stress. During times of stress, you may find yourself turning to food even when you are not hungry. Deal with stress in other ways, perhaps a few deeps breaths or a short walk.
3. Appreciate food. Acknowledge the gift of food and the effort needed to grow and prepare it. Enjoy your food with gratitude.
4. Eat slowly. Eating slowly may help you better recognize your hunger and satiety cues. Try to put your fork down between bites, chew your food well Make each meal last at least 20 minutes.
5. Be mindful about the taste, texture, and smell of food. Savor your food. Notice the flavor, shape, and texture of each bite.
6. Be mindful of portions to enjoy quality, not quantity. When more food is served, we are tempted to eat more. Be mindful of the portion sizes being served on your plate.
7. Be mindful of how hungry you are. External cues such as seeing or smelling food may be signaling you to eat, but are you really hungry?
8. Eat before you get too hungry. When you get too hungry, you may be tempted to make impulsive choices instead of mindful selections.
9. Choose plant-based proteins often such as beans and legumes.
10. Be mindful of your calorie budget. Everyone has a number of calories that can be eaten each day to maintain a healthy weight. Track what you eat and drink. Phone Apps have been shown to be very helpful. Tracking for even a few days can increase your mindfulness of what and how much you are consuming.
11. Determine if the food is calorie-worthy. When it comes to special holiday foods or "sometimes" foods, ask yourself, is this calorie-worthy? If you are going to splurge on a high-calorie food, make sure it is something you really enjoy – then have just a few bites.
12. Take one bite. Follow the one-bite rule when it comes to special foods or desserts. You will not feel deprived from missing out on a favorite food and will not feel guilty for eating too much. The maximum pleasure of eating a food usually comes in the first bite.

MINDLESS EATING

Mindless eating is non-hungry, non-thinking eating. It is the unthinking reaching out for food and snacking on it or gobbling down a meal with problems on your mind or when boozed.

STAY MOTIVATED
Real Reasons Why Diets Fail
- Lack of resolve
- Lack of discipline
- Impatience

Most Listed Excuses to stop Losing Weight
- Lack of time
- Program dissatisfaction

Most usual reactions for excuses
- Not fast enough
- Denial
- Anger
- Rebellion
- Disillusionment
- Burn-out
- Revenge
- Relapse

HOW TO KEEP DIETING
- Weigh every day
- Some "advisors" recommend you don't weigh every day. I think this is as absurd as if an athlete or swimmer wouldn't record their training times
- Put up a Graph
- You will have to make time. Get focused
- Allocate absolutely uninterrupted time each day and week to refine your program and reinforce your efforts
- Dedicate some "Me Time" to recuperate and reorganize
- Most failures are due to lack of willpower and determination
- Next is becoming disappointed or disillusioned at either not losing fast enough or "plateauing" - not losing despite dieting
- Overweight people frequently know more about and are obsessed by food but they just lack will power and persistence
- Never give up. Never give up. Never give up
- Most people who lapse don't or won't change habits
- Be happy with any loss no matter how small

- Do not make goals too hard: Set small initial short-term goals. Don't think "I've only lost a little" but rather "I am losing and heading toward my goal"
- Have small short-term goals rather than one final big one
- Losing weight is slow. It is a marathon
- The more overweight the more unrealistic the expectations
- Discard all preconceptions. This is you. ANY loss is a victory. "Every long journey starts with one small step"
- You will need constant motivation and help. Find a diet partner
- One day at a time. Just today eat less today
- Never feel full. Leave some food on your plate. (Don't worry you won't die - in fact you will live longer)
- Just 100 calories less a day loses weight
- Gain control
- Resolve. Resolve. Resolve. Never give up
- Diets are stressful. You have to keep at it until it becomes your new habit, your new foods your new satiety level (the amount of food that satisfies). This takes at least six weeks
- Find the personal key that best motivates you
    - A photo when you were slimmer
    - A photo of someone you resemble or admire and is lean
    - But no negative photos or measurements that frustrate
    - A graph of your weight, wall planner, waist size
    - NEWTRITION Foods are based on the Mediterranean diet but updated and evidenced to be the healthiest of all and to lose weight. If you stick to these foods and eat less, you will lose weight

Anxiety-Stress provoked snacking:
HALT: Hungry, Angry, Lonely, Tired: Assess whether you're eating out of necessity or any of the HALTs
Eat slowly: Put your fork (or spoon) down between bites.
Think about each mouthful
Try deep breaths before each meal

CHAPTER 4.
MAINTENANCE

Now learn to control your appetite which, with our modern lifestyle, affluence and excess of junk food, is very difficult.

1. Think "Restraint"
2. Think are you actually hungry or just bored, grazing and 'rewarding'
3. Are meals smaller
4. Are there fewer snacks and more formal meals
5. Are there less fat and refined carbohydrates
6. Exercise > 30 mins a day or better still do SIT
7. Look up daily Calorie needs for age, height and sex and don't exceed – in fact eat 600 cals less.
8. Although weight loss is achievable for many adults, weight maintenance is elusive
9. After completing weight loss programs about a third of the weight lost is regained in the following year but an 81% success rate is possible
10. As weight falls metabolism slows, appetite changes – need 100 cals less for every 1kg drop

MAINTENANCE OF WEIGHT LOSS

Post-bariatric surgery behaviors, which would also seem relevant to anyone trying to lose weight, that were significantly linked to weight regain included
- sedentary time
- frequently eating fast food
- eating when full
- eating continuously
- disordered eating such as binge and loss of control eating

Weighing oneself at least once weekly was linked to significantly less weight regain.

Exercise and physical activity, even if just house work or gardening, are especially important.

The latest research has found that Metformin helped maintain long-term weight loss in individuals at risk for type 2 diabetes.

MAINTENANCE MONITORING
1. Are meals smaller?
2. Are you leaving some food on your plate
3. Do you stop before you feel full
4. Non-hungry eating?
5. Intake wrongly estimated – get monitored
6. 'Mindless snacks': More formal meals
7. Weigh daily
8. Are there less fat and refined carbohydrates
9. Is exercise > 30 mins a day or SIT
10. Look up daily Calorie needs for age, height and sex and don't exceed – in fact eat 600 cals less
11. Default value hit – keep going – break through
12. You cannot lose every week. Keep going
13. No unreal expectations: Weight loss is s-l-o-w
14. Ideal loss is 250g a week (that's 13kg a year!)
15. Premenstrual water retention
16. Although weight loss is achievable for many adults, weight maintenance is elusive

TRAPS

Entitlement Justification
* Eating more because you exercise: Dieters ate 79g when they knew they were going to exercise cf 28g when they did not expect to run.
* Too sudden a change with too many changes
* Changing to a diet that you can't stick to forever (? Keto)
* Trying multiple fad diets
* Not increasing physical activity
* Alcohol is an appetite stimulant very high in Empty Calories

Rewards – Comfort
Everybody has their "comfort foods" which we seek when we are stressed, tired, exhausted and such. They donate us a "reward" for all the incredible hard work and problems we have had to grapple with…and make us fat.
No! It's not much of a reward if it makes you fat.
DSD! Do Something Different!

Cravings
Several behavioral studies have demonstrated that denying certain foods, like being on a diet, causes increased craving and motivation for that food. Craving for foods high in fat - this includes many junk foods - is an important part of obesity and binge eating. When trying to lose weight people often strive to avoid fatty foods, which ironically increases motivation and craving

for these foods and can lead to overeating. Even worse, the longer someone abstains from fatty foods, the greater the cravings. Don't ban your cravings all together – you'll only miss them more and they can become an obsession and you then pig out. Have some but try and minimize.

Lower craving has ben linked to more exposure to green spaces. Having access to a garden or allotment was associated with both lower craving strength and frequency, while residential views incorporating more than 25% greenspace evoked similar responses.

DISILLUSIONMENT: Plan
- Re-list the reasons you want to lose
- Realistic goals 250g/wk
- Look at this list: Read this book
- Reorganize your plan, start again, get help
- Enjoy gaining control and getting fit
- Be Positive: You may not be losing but getting fit

NOT LOSING
- Intake wrongly estimated – get monitored
- Default value hit – keep going – break through
- You cannot lose every week. Keep going
- No unreal expectations: Weight loss is s-l-o-w
- Ideal loss is 250g a week (that's 13kg a year!)
- Premenstrual water retention
- Enjoy gaining control and getting fit.
- Don't be discouraged by setbacks. Push through
- Learn to read labels. 'Sugar' is disguised as alternate names
- Simplest is to avoid all packaged or wrapped food
- Mother Hubbard (bare cupboard): Don't buy it you can't eat it
- No fat patient thinks they eat to excess. Their satiety index is set high
- They honestly don't know they are eating more than they need
- There was never a fat prisoner of war but our genes or our microbiome haven't changed
- Fat owners have fat dogs
- Eating less is 85% of weight loss, 15% is exercise
- But you need BOTH!
- The exercise needed to burn off food calories is far too great to correlate with actual weight lost. There must be some other mechanism at work especially with Resistance Weight Training
- Exercise make you more efficient at metabolizing food and burning off
- Calories and it also reduces mortality
- But you can eat smarter: Women who ate more fruit and vegetables which were water-rich, lost 33% more weight in the first 6 months compared to those on a low-fat diet. Despite the fact they ate more food by weight, they actually ate less Calories
- Eat high volume, high nutrition. Water content is the key

HINTS, TRICKS and GOOD ADVICE

Habits of The Most Successful Slimmers
These habits may not be obvious as their practitioners seldom make a big issue as to their behavior(s), or it has been so entrenched that it is familiar second nature and people accept this as their normal manner of conduct e.g. "(S)he eats like a bird" of persons we all know as not eating much and we accept their actions as 'just being them'. These twelve daily habits define some of the best-looking people:

1. Total ruthless dedication to their plan
2. Daily control and continuance. Never give up
3. Emancipation not deprivation
4. The best foods (Newtrition Super-Mediterranean)
5. Never feeling full. Always leaving something on the plate
6. Interest in health. Pride in appearance
7. Aerobic and Resistance exercise
8. Always alternatives to eating (exercise or occupation)
9. Portion control
10. No processed foods. No sugar or refined carbs
11. Dedication, Determination, Discipline, Resolve and Restraint
12. Anti-Disillusionment strategies

MORE HINTS
- Re-set your volume control. Eat smaller portions. Think thin: Think small.
- While calories and volume are not the same, they are if you eat high nutrition foods. If we eat greater volumes, they fill us more
- Portion Distortion: From 1960 - 2012 portion sizes increased > x 10 times for coke and 100 cals for fries, hamburgers
- Only 20 more cals a day gains weight; 100 cals extra a day to become obese
- People do not notice an extra 1000cals a day. "Insensible eating" Monitor!
- Eat with someone who eats small amounts – social modeling
- Never eat everything on your plate. Leave a third. Never eat until you feel 'full'
- Eat less, just two days a week
- Intermittent fasts – 600cal days x 2 a week. Otherwise, rest of week, eat as before
- Eating 600 calories a day less for men from 2,400 to 1,800 calories gave better results (fat 2.3 vs 1.3% in six months)
- Think more vegetarian who are the slimmest people but not in twin studies (one eats meat). So, Lifestyle also helps.

- Stick to the Newtrition Foods (emphasizing vegetarian). Don't worry about % of protein, carbohydrate or fats
- Otherwise measure Cals av = < 1800/ day men, <1,500 Cals women
- This with a nearly vegetarian/fish diet, is the secret of most world's longest living people
- Get your mind made up, determined and set. No excuses, no stress, no competing interests
- Ensure some 'my time' to get away, review and plan each week
- Get help. Enlist a partner to monitor and support
- Avoid the 'Supermarket' and processed foods
- Compensate for junk by buying the best as a substitution reward
- Identify hi-Cal junk foods and avoid
- Whole fruit and small half-hand-full nuts for snacks
- Exercise - the type doesn't matter (SIT best) but you must also eat less.
- Eating less is far more efficient than exercise
- Beware the exercise 'Entitlement Trap' that exercise 'justifies' more food.
- Exercise can weaken self-control
- No unearned 'rewards'. Treats must be earned e.g. after a sustained minimum 3 kg loss.
- But then resume eating less
- To lose - No booze
- Measure waist circumference
- Weigh daily
- Diet diary-Phone App excellent help – but record everything
- Everyone falls off the wagon, gets disillusioned, but this should be a key to get going again
- You will hit the wall and feel lousy at six weeks or 10% weight loss. Be warned! Continue! Increase exercise.
- Your body will hit its default values - the weights you were stuck on as you gained and will resist change. Continue
- No unreal expectations. Don't feel sorry for yourself – the lean also have to work at it too
- Think long term: 250 g loss a week = 13 kg a year = 28.6lb or 2 stone a year. (Would you like to gain that?)
- Put up a photo of someone you want to look like

- Don't shop when hungry – if you don't buy it you can't eat it. Remember Mother Hubbard – she was lean
- Identify triggers or cravings – make plans to avoid. Identify non-hungry eating
- People who don't lose underestimate the food they eat by 47% to 67% and overestimate activity by 40% to 51%
- Fat people unconsciously snack.
- Don't open the fridge and graze. Hide snacks lower shelf at back
- Make eating formal, pleasant and slow. No mindless snacking in front of TV.
- Minimize restaurants and Takeaways.
- People ate twice the amount of M&Ms if they were labeled 'lite'.
- Don't believe "Lite, No sugar, Sugar reduced, Low Fat"
- Don't start unless and until you are absolutely resolved and committed with no excuses
- Restricting dietary fat can lead to greater body fat loss than carb restriction
- Clear the kitchen bench of everything but the fruit bowl
- Catch the bus or train. Use the stairs.
- Vegans have the lowest BMI, then vegetarians but not by much in identical twin studies where one ate meat there was only a 1.5kg difference. Vegans usually have a stricter Lifestyle.
- People keenly interested food are usually interested in their health and therefore their weight
- When selecting foods in a sequence (e.g., at a buffet), individuals are influenced by the first item they see and tend to make their subsequent food choices on the basis of this first item. This can be utilized. When an indulgent dish is the first item, lower-calorie dishes are subsequently chosen, and overall caloric consumption is lower and vice versa.
- Medicine has vogues and fads, and the latest vogue is the Gut microbiome or microbes. While this plays as yet an unknown but important place, it is not the complete multifactorial answer
- Scientists found that sweet, bitter, and other taste receptors found in the mouth also exist in the gut — so the gut tastes food after it is consumed. Carbohydrates can thus be preferred.
- We can blame our genes, we can blame our gut but, if we are to lose weight, we have to eat smaller amounts (less calories) and avoid processed foods

CHAPTER 5.
THE BENEFITS of WEIGHT CONTROL

There are risks being overweight even If Fit

Calorie Restriction Increases Longevity

Estimated Benefits of 10% Weight Loss

- BP: Fall of 10 mm in blood pressure if hypertense
- Diabetes: Reversal of Type 2
- Fall of up to 50% in fasting glucose in newly diagnosed patients.
- 3 to 4yr increased life span
  Journal of the American College of Cardiology September 11, 2017
- 30% fall in fasting insulins
- 30% increase in insulin sensitivity
- 40% - 60% fall in incidence of diabetes
- Lipids - improve
  - Fall 10% in total cholesterol
  - Fall 15% in LDL (bad) cholesterol
  - Fall 30% in triglycerides
  - Rise 8% in HDL (good) cholesterol
- Mortality
  - 20% fall in all-cause mortality
  - 30% fall in deaths related to diabetes
  - 40% fall in deaths related to obesity

CONSEQUENCES OF OVERWEIGHT / OBESITY

Medical
Diabetes 2
Metabolic Syndrome
CardioVascular: Hypertension, heart attacks, Coronary Heart Disease, heart Failure, atrial fibrillation, strokes, Varicose veins, piles, Dyslipidaemia (cholesterol / triglycerides)
Cancer
Breathlessness, fatigue, lassitude, aches, pains, indigestion, heat intolerance
Sleep Apnoea, snoring, somnolence, poor concentration
Gallstones, Gall Bladder Disease, Cirrhosis

Increased morbidity and mortality – all causes
Osteoarthritis, neck problems / spondylosis – facet locking, Low back pain
Hyperuricaemia and gout
Pregnancy Complications, Foetal defects, Impaired fertility / Polycystic ovary syndrome, menstrual disorders
Impotence
Hirsutism
Anesthetic risk
Depression, low self-esteem, lowered confidence, personality changes
Excess sweat, rashes, intertrigo, thrush, chafing, hygiene problems
Neglected feet

Social
Psychological
Social Penalties
Discrimination – less likely to be hired or promoted
Obese employees have twice the rate of absenteeism & compensation claims
For every 1 kg excess employees are paid $500 p.a. less
Social derision; the butt of jokes
Embarrassment with seating, crowds

SLIM 4 LIFE KEY ESSENTIALS

1. Commit- Make Time – Resolve
2. Phone App – record everything - 10% loss
3. Chew slowly – up to 42% loss
4. Wait 20 minutes to abate hunger
5. Eat less. Select diet that works for you
6. No snacks after dinner
7. Discard all processed foods. Avoid eating any
8. Newtrition Super-Mediterranean Foods
9. Plan Ahead
10. Identify Triggers
11. Change bad Habits for better Lifestyles
12. Weigh daily. Measure waist monthly.
13. Smaller portions / plates
14. When target met then for any gain starve next day until lost
15. Put up a photo of a shape you'd like to be
16. Only a fruit bowl on the kitchen bench
17. 40 seconds three times a week exercise bike
18. Resistance training
19. Don't eat more because you exercise
20. Water boarding (fill up on water)
21. Hi-volume, lo-cal foods
22. Take the stairs
23. Waists: Men < 102 cm. Women < 88 cm
24. Any fat hanging over your belt is bad

Snacks – foods that fill more

Based on a 1990s Sydney University study where white bread was rated as the 100th.

i. Potatoes
ii. White fish
iii. Porridge
iv. Oranges
v. Apples
vi. Pasta brown
vii. Beef steak
viii. Baked Beans
ix. Grapes
x. Bread wholemeal
xi. Popcorn
xii. All Bran
xiii. Eggs
xiv. Cheese
xv. Rice white
xvi. Lentils

Slim 4 Life recommends chilled grapes or apples and potatoes if cold (_small amount_)
Foods with high water content: Fill you more with less calories
Cucumbers and iceberg lettuce 96% water.
Celery, tomatoes and zucchini: 95-94% water
Broccoli, cabbage, cauliflower, capsicums, spinach: 93-91% water
Finally, it has been observed that 'the price of freedom is eternal vigilance'.
This too, is the price of keeping ourselves slim and trim.

BOOK 5

EXERCISES
&
PHYSICAL
ACTIVITIES

Middle aged and older adults, including those with cardiovascular disease and cancer, can gain substantial longevity benefits by becoming more physically active, irrespective of past physical activity levels and established risk factors. Considerable population health impacts can be attained with consistent engagement in physical activity during mid to late life.

At the population level, meeting and maintaining at least the minimum physical activity recommendations would potentially prevent 46% of deaths associated with physical inactivity.

Physical activity trajectories and mortality: population based cohort study
BMJ 2019; 365 doi: https://doi.org/10.1136/bmj.l2323 (Published 26 June 2019)
Cite this as: BMJ 2019;365:l2323

Lack of physical activity accounts for
- 22% of coronary heart disease
- 22% of colon cancer
- 18% of osteoporotic fractures
- 12% percent of diabetes and hypertension
- 5% of breast cancer

INTRODUCTION

Lack of exercise is responsible for twice as many early deaths as obesity. There is nothing else that can influence as many organ systems in a positive manner as can physical activity.
Age changes are mostly attributable to inactivity. Optimum ageing necessitates exercise. Staying physically active can buy extra years of function compared to sedentary people.

This does not mean you have to join a gym, get a personal trainer or such. What follows are sensible, achievable subtle life-style modifications from just getting the sedentary to stand more, which has profound benefits, to activities and exercises for each age group who want to do more.

This is not a book for those who already exercise but even so, there are some detailed revelations included, which may fine-tune their regimes.
It is mainly a book, like Slim 4 Life, for those of us who have insidiously slipped into bad habits and in this case, become more sedentary. It is also for those who have never really started.

But, as above, it is absolutely vital you now do so…or die sooner than you should.

The main aim is to increase our exercise through every-day normal activities and not having to enroll in a gym, buy expensive equipment (well just one if you can but there's no real need).

Exercise doesn't lose much weight per se, but it does tune-up our whole metabolic system and optimizes our health.

The fattest people on Earth are the Pima Indians of Arizona who are greatly affected by diabetes, kidney failure and heart disease. They inherited a financial bonanza when they got Casino gambling rights. They don't work much, have drive-thru fast food outlets with plenty of deep-fried foods and are obese.

Whereas the same tribe, with the same identical genes and therefore the same predisposition to such illnesses and premature deaths, were separated by a flood of the Colorado River some 600 years ago and settled in Mexico. They are poor. The children walk at least 2 miles to school, the men till the fields with horse and plough and they eat home-made tortillas and fresh food. They are not obese, do not suffer the consequent illnesses and live longer.

My generation ran and ran and ran as kids and played sport. Today when I examine 11 to 16 year-old boys I see many have "man-boobs" and when I ask them if they play sport it is very rare that one says "yes". But they all have Smart phones and Video Games.

Better public transport, owning our own cars and labour-saving devices, from back-hoes to pre-mixed concrete, makes manual labour a distant memory. Few of us grow our own vegies.

On top of this we have processed junk-food available 24 hours a day, seven days a week and home delivered such that even getting up to pay for the pizza is an effort - especially when we have the ultimate labour-saver, the TV Remote.

It has become so perverse that those young people who want to get fit have to join a gym and can't realise how every day activities can be as an efficient work-out.

Then there are the mandatory uniforms: The Mamils - Middle Age Men In Lycra - on their bikes, the girls in lycra or athletic bras with, as one observer noted, "fixed smiles betraying the incredible loneliness and disassociation of such places' (perhaps Tinder will replace them). And then there are the (very) expensive shoes for which actual medical research can find no benefits - at least not those claimed by the manufacturers. So they are fashion statements too.

But, if it gets them out there and exercising they are to be lauded.

There is much we can do in our normal everyday activities. You will see how slow walking is associated with a shorter lifespan as is a weaker hand-grip and sitting down too much.

Now I can't claim to be a long liver but at 78 years old I still work 10 hours a day at medicine (12 hour days last week in fact), work around our farm and walk faster than all the people in the city mall when I go to get a hair-cut... and I don't do this deliberately: I simply can't get over how people dawdle. ("Dawdle and die" perhaps?).

And so we come to what exercises then are most suitable for us, at our age and maybe carrying some condition such as osteoarthritis of the hips or knees.

But whatever, as you will see, "exercise is arguably the best thing you can do for your health".

What I have done is researched the best, beneficial exercises for all ages. This is no six-pack Fitness Instructor urging, but the trials, programs and results of the world's best studies. When you read the chapter on "Benefits" you will be staggered and if this isn't enough to get you going, nothing, I know, will.

People have never been healthier and lived longer as when there was food rationing as in World War 1 and 2, the Dust Bowl Famines of the USA in the 30s and the Cuban embargo.

The lean live longest. Perhaps the observations of the lean, long-living Okinawans may be a good concept and premise for us to adopt: "Never feel full. Always leave something on your plate".

CHAPTER 1.
THE BEST MEDICINE

THE BEST MEDICINE

Lack of exercise responsible for twice as many early deaths as obesity.

There is nothing else that can influence as many organ systems in a positive manner as can physical activity.

Age changes are mostly attributable to inactivity. Optimum ageing necessitates exercise. Inevitably, our bodies will experience declines with age, but staying physically active can buy extra years of function compared to sedentary people.

Who Benefits From This Book
This is much more than a book of exercises or fitness guide by some incredible athlete or trainer - it is a *medical* book for you to find out just what exercises donate the best benefits to you for your health and longevity and why you should be doing them.

Exercise is incredibly beneficial to our health yet progressively difficult to achieve in this increasingly labour saving, drive-thru, TV Remote, sedentary life.

The committed athlete and even those who are devoted walkers, gym-junkies or work-out devotees will have their own routines by which they swear. This book is not to alter their regimes but even they may find some valuable information.

The Goldilocks Problem – What Exercise Is 'Just Right'
While Live Longest covers most medically evidenced, beneficial exercise regimes from basic to advanced, from just Walking through to HIIT (High Intensity Interval Training) and HICT (High Intensity Circuit Training), two regimes are recommended as they uniquely can be adapted and adopted by the old and frail right through to the elite athlete.

The Two Recommended Regimes
They two are a 40 second SIT (Sprint Interval Training) with Resistance Weights and HIIPA (High Intensity Incidental Physical Activity) which

is an add on to optimise and maximise normal daily activities. SIT does require an Exercise Bike but there is no other equipment really necessary and the convenience, time savings and lack of knee damage make it a well worthwhile purchase. But there are other substitutes if you can't afford one.

What this book sets out to do is inform you as to:
1. The best exercises - don't waste your time: Find the one(s) that suit you best
2. The best exercises for your age
3. The benefits to be derived

This book will cover the best exercises for all ages and conditions. A 70 year-old is obviously not going to do what a fit 20 year old can do, and an unfit 20 year old won't be able to do what a fit 20 year old can do.

It is important that you start gently.

The research and trials as to what advanced regimes provide the greatest benefit is provided for those able to achieve thejm.

It is thought that a dose-response exists for physical activity and health benefits: The more and more intense the greater the benefits. This improves Glucose tolerance and better metabolic gain. But this may be modified as a Danish 12-year prospective study found that slow and moderate joggers live longer than both their fast-paced and sedentary peers and those who exercised strenuously had similar all-cause mortality to those who didn't jog at all.

The modern approach is for HIIT- High Intensity Interval Training but this is too intense for most.

But do something!

Anything!

Get just getting up to stand regularly has been found to have great benefits.

Exercise Liberates EVs to Signal the Whole Body
Following a 1-hr bout of cycling exercise in healthy humans, there is an increase in the circulation of over 300 proteins, with a notable enrichment of several classes of proteins that compose exosomes and small vesicles. These EVs liberated by exercise have a propensity to localize in the liver and can transfer their protein cargo. In addition several novel candidate myokines, are released into circulation independently of classical secretion. These identify a new paradigm by which tissue crosstalk during exercise can exert systemic biological effects.

CHAPTER 2.
DEFINITIONS

I hope this clarifies the jargon of today, there seems to be as many abbreviations as there are gyms, but also to identify the different types of exercises and their benefits.

Physical Activity:
any movement that burns calories such as mowing lawns, walking upstairs, making the bed, walking the dog

Exercise:
Structured physical activity with a series of repetitive movements designed to strengthen or develop part of your body and improve cardiovascular fitness eg walking, swimming, bicycling

Moderate activity: such as gentle swimming, housework, social tennis
Vigorous activity: such as jogging, aerobics or competitive tennis

Anaerobic: Not needing oxygen. Strength or Resistance Training

Aerobic: Means using oxygen. Cardiovascular - Respiratory Fitness

Balance: An even distribution of weight enabling the person to remain upright and steady.

Physiology: The body's internal processes.

Sarcopenia: The loss of skeletal muscle mass and strength as a result of ageing.

Exercise grades
- Low: Almost completely inactive (reading, watching TV or minor physical activity)
- Moderate: Some physical activity for > 4 hrs a week of cycling, light gardening or walking
- High: Vigorous physical activity > 3 hrs / wk (such as running, swimming, heavy gardening, competitive sports)

New Intensity Exercises and Nomenclature

The exercise 'Industry' has now come up with numerous confusing permutations and combinations often referred to by their abbreviations but without the following explanations:

HIIT: High Intensity Interval Training - short bursts of demanding exercise interspersed with short rests

HHIT: Home HIIT

HIRT: the same, but with resistance training

HIFT: the functional version, designed to prepare you for any movement

MCIT or MOD: Moderate-Intensity Continuous Training

LISS: Low-Intensity Steady-State exercise, even a gentle stroll can now, technically, count and be considered a productive fat-loss session

HIIPA: High Intensity Incidental Physical Activity. Now touted as a simple way to push your body into healthy adaptation without disrupting your daily schedule.

Changes recommended include using the stairs, carrying the shopping for 100 to 200 meters, walk at a pace to that you find it hard to speak – puff.

SIT: Sprint Interval Training

LPA: light physical activity

MVPA: Moderate to vigorous physical activity

MEASUREMENT: METS

Intensity of Exercise
* Most exercise machines today measure exercise in METs
* **1 MET or Metabolic Equivalent Task = 1 Cal body wt / hr**
* = energy expended by sitting quietly & breathing or the oxygen uptake when at rest
* = 3.5 ml O2 /kg/min
* Vigorous activity = 6 METS or greater. eg: jogging, running, rowing, swimming, tennis, squash

Don't Worry About METS:
Most exercise machines give MET readouts, but Fitness Instructors largely ignore them. They are, after all, *just a measure* of what you are doing and if you are sweating and doing vigorous exercise this is enough and all you have to do is keep, either a time, distance or weights record, and make sure you sweat and puff a little.

If you have a machine that gives a MET or other read out it is a record and motivator.

MET scores range from 1 to 12, where 1 is considered the equivalent of sitting on the couch, 3 aligns with walking, 7 with jogging, 10 with jumping rope and 12 with sprinting.

Each 1 MET increase in activity for overweight women was independently associated with an 8% decrease in the risk of adverse major CVS events.

Formula to Work Out Your MET level and relevance to Death Rate

Predicted exercise capacity women	=	14.7 minus (0.13 x age)
eg 50 year old	=	14.7 – (0.13 x 50 = 6.5)
14.7 – 6.5	=	8.2 METs = 100%
85%	=	6.97
Predicted exercise capacity for men	=	14.7 minus (0.11 x age)
eg 50 year old man	=	14.7 – (0.11 x 50 = 5.5)
14.7 – 5.5	=	9.2 METs = 100%
85%	=	7.82

Exercise machines can automatically calculate METS
<85% of this predicted value doubles the death rate

CHAPTER 3.
EXERCISE TYPES

    A. ANAEROBIC: Strength or Resistance Training
    B. AEROBIC: Cardiovascular - Respiratory Fitness
    C. BALANCE, FLEXIBILITY and STRETCHING

A. ANAEROBIC: STRENGTH / RESISTANCE TRAINING

Anaerobic exercise comprises brief, strength-based activities, such as sprinting or bodybuilding, whereas aerobic exercise is centered around endurance activities, such as marathon running or long-distance cycling. However, the early stage of all exercise is anaerobic. Anaerobic exercise cause lactate (lactic acid) to form. It promotes strength, speed and power and is used by body builders to build muscle mass. Muscle energy systems trained using anaerobic exercise develop differently compared to aerobic exercise, leading to greater performance in short duration, high intensity activities, which last from mere seconds to up to about 2 minutes. Modern exercise science shows that working with weights—whether that weight is a light dumbbell or your own body—may be the best exercise for lifelong physical function and fitness.

* Builds stronger leaner muscles to increase metabolism, support & protect joints, promotes balance & coordination, improve posture, slows bone loss, cuts injury, promotes energy
* People lose 10% of lean muscle each decade after 30
* If this muscle loss is not replaced, fat increases
* Weight training is recommended for all over 50 years

Benefits
1. Decreased body fat
2. Increased lean body mass
3. Increased strength
4. Increased bone mineral density (less osteoporosis)
5. Better Blood Glucose metabolism
6. Increased BMR (metabolism)
7. Increased sub-maximal (aerobic) fitness
8. Improves mood & cognitive function in elderly
9. However, Intensive weight training stiffened the arteries in healthy men and thus resistance training should proceed cautiously in those at risk

Results
- 113.0% improvement in strength
- 11.3% improvement in walking speed
- 28.4% improvement in stair climbing power

Weight Training Definitions
- Set = a specific exercise at a specific resistance for a set number of times
- Repetition = repeating the one exercise
- Maximum = heaviest weight for 1 repetition maintaining good technique

Regime: SORPS (Specificity, Overload, Repetition, Progression, Stretching)
Specificity
> Different muscle groups each day. Never exercise the same muscle group 2 days straight

Overload (Most people don't achieve this)
> 80% of max. weight you can lift for each muscle group
> (Elderly: 30-40% upper, 50-60% lower)

Repetition
> 3 sets of 8 to 10 (15) lifts (20 mins)
> Lift to fatigue. Slowly increase weight = 'maxing out'
> Most injuries are from trying to max out too early

Progression
> Re-measure maximum weight each month

Stretching

Efficiency: No rest between sets by exercising another muscle mass (upper-lower), a 40 min workout reduces to 20 min. Note: Weight training effects last 48 hours.

Best Resistance Activities
* Swimming / cycling = resistance training (but with some aerobic - breathlessness - input
* Cycling not only keeps you mentally alert, but requires the vigorous use of many of the body's key systems, such as muscles, heart and lungs which are needed for maintaining health and for reducing the risks associated with numerous diseases but may lead to osteoporosis, especially in women, as there is no weight bearing
* Swimming, however, is arguably the best exercise as it halves the body weight thereby protecting the joints (other than the shoulder joint if undue excess) while using most muscle masses
* Weights, of course, are very good but caution should be taken with overhead exercises as these frequently result in shoulder capsule injuries. Best not done after 45 yrs.

What is strength training?
Strength training encompasses any of the following:
* Free weights, such as barbells and dumbbells
* Ankle cuffs and vests containing different amounts of weight
* Resistance (elastic) bands of varying length and tension that you flex using your arms and legs
* Exercises that use your body weight to create resistance against gravity.

How much do you need?
A beginner's strength-building workout takes as little as 20 minutes, and you won't need to grunt, strain, or sweat like a cartoon bodybuilder, either. The key is developing a well-rounded program, performing the exercises with good form, and being consistent. You will experience noticeable gains in strength within four to eight weeks.

B. AEROBIC:
CARDIO VASCULAR - RESPIRATORY FITNESS

Walking / Aerobics (endurance exercise):
Aerobic or cardio exercise is that of low to high intensity that 'sucks it in'. Light-to-moderate intensity aerobic exercises can be performed for extended periods of time. Any activity lasting longer than about two minutes has a large aerobic metabolic component. Aerobic exercise includes lower intensity activities performed for longer periods of time such as walking, jogging, long slow runs, rowing, swimming and cycling. These require a great deal of oxygen to generate the energy needed for prolonged (aerobic) exercise.

These exercises involve repeated contractions of large muscle groups (e.g. arms & legs) but not speed as in sprinting. Increase and improved breathing & heart rate, increased endurance.

Benefits
       How much exercise - a graded response:
* 12 miles jogging per week resulted in beneficial changes to the lipid profile
* 20 miles per week resulted in more pronounced changes and were required to produce increases in good HDL Cholesterol levels
* Women progressively more active had 11, 19, 22 & 28% fewer total CVS events. The most active (28%) walked @ 3mph for 1 hour each day or 23.4 hrs/wk

Heart Rate

Aerobic exercise is for heart-lung fitness and optimum achievable heart rate should be known. You should not exceed these.

Two Systems according to age group:
1. Target
2. BORG Perceived Exertion

1. Target Heart Rate:
Best for Young

AGE	Max HR 100%	Target HR 70 – 85%
20	200	140 – 170
25	195	136 - 166
30	190	133 – 161
35	185	129 – 157
40	180	126 – 153
45	175	122 - 149
50	170	119 – 144
55	165	115 – 140
60	160	108 – 136
65	155	108 – 132
70	150	– 127

2. BORG RPE Rating of Perceived Exertion:
Best for elderly. Self rate: Stay at 12 to 14.

Rating		Interpretation
6		Rest
7		Very, very light
8		-
9		Very light
10		-
11		Fairly light
12		-
13	'The Zone'	Somewhat hard
14		-
15		Hard
16		-
17		Very hard
18		-
19		Very, very hard
20		Maximum effort

C. BALANCE, FLEXIBILITY and STRETCHING
- Balance starts to decline at 40
- Helps maintain the ideal range of bending and flexibility around joints.
- Maximises the motion about a joint; helps prevent injury and pain (arthritis).
- Balance helps prevent falls and injuries - especially later in life
- Strength training can increase the range of joint motion in elderly and inactive improving function and reducing accidents
- 10 resistance exercises of major muscle groups significantly improved sit & reach, elbow, shoulder & knee flexion and hip extension

The Core
- The term for the body's centre of gravity ie the area around the trunk & pelvis
- Good muscle tone and synchronisation of the core is now recognised as fundamental to good posture, low back and pelvic floor problem prevention
- The core provides stabilisation necessary from lifting weights to jogging to tennis
- Core strengthening involves all overlapping muscles of the abdomen and trunk

Stretching
- Despite Sports gurus recommending and advocating stretching, no medical benefit has been found

Home-Based Exercise Program Prevented Falls Among Elders
In a Canadian study, the incidence of major falls dropped by about one third.

CHAPTER 4.
PLANNING

Pre-Start

Medical - get a check-up first -
Assess your fitness level. Do basic measurements:
- Weight
- Waist
- Distance
- Time

Mental:
- Make commitment / resolve - as if an appointment to keep
- Select exercises to suit and you enjoy
- Allocate time(s) - design program - be flexible - avoid sun
- Set realistic goals - this is not a race - but logical progress

Commit
- Make this an important appointment you cannot break
- Have back-up contingency Plan B
- Have spare kit
- Factor in traffic delays etc
- If outdoors, have indoor alternative for bad weather

Equipment / clothes / gear as necessary
- Shoes
- Track-suit / sun-proof Hat / sunglasses / suncream
- Weights (sand bags / socks), Rubber bands
- Exercise Bike if you can

Keep a record:
- Start slowly - aim for 30 min a day 5 days a week. Keep at it
- Slowly improve viz: more steps, faster times, further distances, increased weights

CHAPTER 5.
MOTIVATION

Developing the Habit

It's not what you do, but how you get yourself to exercise that matters. Developing any habit -- good or bad -- starts with a routine, and exercise is no exception. The trick is making exercise a habit that is hard to break.

Focus on cues that trigger you do it. It is this instigation habit, the triggers that prompt people to automatically go for their walk/jog, lift weighs, that increases exercise frequency.

It may take a month or longer of repeated behavior before a cue reliably and automatically triggers a behavior; sticking with the same time of day helps initially.

As you lose weight your Metabolic Rate falls and you have to do more

Researched Motivators
Immediate Objective
Identify what you most want from exercise *now*.
Quality of Life: Less stress, more energy and coping better preferred to health improvement

Set and measure goals
Setting specific, measurable goals such as a greater distance or improved times and weights but must be realistic and practical

Plan
Make it a regular appointment you *must* keep. Ensure time set aside. Have back-up contingencies. Plan B, extra kit, traffic snarl-delays, alternate emergency time.

Duration
Everyone is time poor today. Make it short: Sit or Home HIT

Entertain yourself
Fitness apps (e.g. The Walk and Zombies, Run!), books on tape, podcasts, movies or TV shows, can reduce boredom.

Companion
Motivation is boosted by up to 85% when others around you are *slightly*, but not much, better than you.

Pay Yourself
We love receiving money, but we hate losing it even more. This is known as "loss aversion". Pay yourself upfront, say $50 a month, and deduct $5 for every session missed.

Tips
- Just do it.
- The more you think about it the less you feel like doing it
- Thinking about exercising undermines resolve
- Become self-motivated - don't depend on anyone else
- Make exercise an important priority
- Make it a routine and a habit
- Select best time: Early morning, after work, evening.
- No commitment that can make you miss or cancel
- Fit exercise into your daily routines not vice versa
- Pick activities you like to do. Walk the dog. Get a dog
- Gyms and personal trainers only if you can't motivate yourself
- Choose activity that suits you. Solitude / group
- Get support. Join a class - 81% continue on cf 61% who drop out without support
- A companion. or Walking/ Gym / Swimming Squad makes excuses difficult & pushes you
- Socialise, have fun
- Mix it up - change routines / exercise type / variety. New Routes
- Small bursts
- Pedometers give a sense of control and motivation (but not intensity)
- Have a goal - set goals
- Ensure adequate sleep and contented mood
- Shorten workouts – SIT or 6x5 x 30 min brisk walking or 12,000 steps. But even 4000 to 5000 steps were associated with benefit, with no evidence of benefit for more than 7500 steps daily
- Use distractions: Music, exercise apps, videos, podcasts, radio. Get an I-Pod / Ear piece radio
- For people insufficiently active, music can not only help them work harder physically during HIIT but it can also help them enjoy HIIT more.
- Motivational music has the power to enhance people's HIIT workouts, it may ultimately give people an extra boost to try HIIT again in the future.

- Set precise 4 week goals e.g. Lengthen distance, decrease time, increased weights
- Plan ahead and stick to it
- Reward for targets eg I-pod; Pay yourself
- Contract eg slice of cake = 2 hrs shopping / walking
- Be satisfied: Think how it is benefiting you. Focus on benefits
- Have a contingency back-up. Plan B. A spare set of exercise gear reduces your excuses.
- Use ski poles if running e.g. cross country - burn 20% more Cals
- Climbing a flight of stairs x 1 to x 5 a day increased oxygen consumption by 17% and decreased LDL by 8%
- Dog owners spent close to 300 minutes each week walking with their dogs, about 200 more minutes of walking than people without dogs.

But _do something_ - anything is better than nothing
Just do it. The more you think about it the less you feel like doing it

---

Special Groups: Arthritis etc: Low impact – Hydrotherapy / Swimming

CHAPTER 6.
HIIPA

High Intensity Incidental Physical Activity

These activities are where you can start immediately and every day from now on.
HIIPA uses normal lifestyle practices without disrupting your daily schedule to get fit.
The idea is to optimize and maximise routines e.g. walk faster, walk longer distances, taker the stairs, get up and down from your desk or TV more frequently, use shopping as weights but, above all, don't resent any of these but rather embrace them and seek other ways you can incorporate exercise into your daily life.

Daily activities / necessities you can crank-up:
- Walk to work - or even 2 blocks – walk fast – puff
- Walk briskly everywhere every time
- Always walk if < 1 km
- Walk the dog - you lead!
- Gardening - do more
- Take the stairs
- Sports you love - regular commitment
- No drive thrus
- No remotes
- Have walking breaks.
- 2,000 steps / day (15 min) controls weight
- Take several trips to unload your groceries. Use them as weights ("curls")
- Regular exercise in men aged 45 - 75
- Exercise reduced waist and body fat while weight remained the same
- Insulin response to glucose improved by 16%
- This may help prevent Diabetes 2 / metabolic syndrome
- Kids who cycle to school are 8% fitter than those who walk.
- 10 to 15 minutes of cycling twice a day is enough to increase kid's aerobic fitness.

Risks
- There are significant risks with sudden unaccustomed exercise
- So start slowly and have a graded plan
- Cease if distressed in any way
- There is also the risk of getting 'hooked' on the endo-morphine high as with the Female Athlete Triad / compulsive trainers

Benefits

Population Group	Type and Amount of Ativities	Observed Benefit
10,269 Harvard alumni	Walking at least 9 miles a week	22% lower death rate
	Climbing at least 55 flights of stairs a week	33% lower death rate
836 residents of King County, Washington	Gardening at least 1 hour/week	66% lower risk for sudden cardiac death
	Walking at least 1 hour/week	73% lower risk for sudden cardiac death
1453 middle-aged Finnish men	At least 2.2 hours of leisure time activity a week	69% lower risk for heart attack
4484 Icelandic men aged 45-80	Spending at least 43 minutes a day on leisure time physical activity after age 40	16% lower risk for stroke
73,743 American women aged 50-79	Walking for at least 2.5 hours per week	30% lower risk for cardiovascular events
44,452 American male health professionals	Walking at least 30 minutes/day	18% lower risk for coronary artery disease
39,372 American female health professionals	Walking at least 1 hour/week	51% lower risk for coronary artery disease
72,488 American female nurses	Walking at least 3 hours/week	35% lower risk for heart attack and cardiac death
		34% lower risk for stroke
30,640 Danish men and women aged 20-93	Spending 2-4 hours/week on light leisure time activity	32% lower mortality rate
4311 British men aged 40-59	Performing light-to-moderate physical activity	35% to 39% lower mortality rate
1404 female residents of Framingham, Massachusetts	Performing moderate physical activity	37% lower mortality rate
802 Dutch men, aged 64-84	Walking or biking at least 1 hour/week	29% lower mortality rate
707 retired Hawaiian men, aged 61-81	Walking at least 2 miles/day	50% lower mortality rate
9518 older American women	Walking up to 10 miles/week	29% lower mortality rate

Population Group	Type and Amount of Ativities	Observed Benefit
229 postmenopausal American women	Walking 1 mile/day or more (a 10-year randomized clinical trial)	82% lower risk for heart disease
7951 pairs of Finnish twins	Exercising at least 30 minutes on at least 6 days/month	43% lower mortality rate
6017 Japanese men, aged 35-60	Walking (to work) for 21 minutes or more on work days	29% lower risk of developing hypertension
1645 Americans aged 65 and older	Walking more than 4 hours/week	27% lower mortality rate
		31% lower risk for hospitalization for heart disease
3206 Swedish men and women aged 65 and older	Performing physical activity at least once a week	40% lower mortality rate
3316 Finnish men and women with type 2 diabetes	Performing moderate leisure time physical activity	18% lower mortality rate
1204 Swedish men and 550 women aged 45-70	Walking or performing demanding household work	54% (men) and 84% (women), lowers risk for heart attacks
2229 European men and women aged 70-90	Performing moderate physical activity	37% lower mortality rate

Cardio Metabolic Exercise (CME) Points for Selected Activities

Activity	Pace	Duration	CME Points
Carpentry	Moderate	30 minutes	100
Cleaning	Heavy	30 minutes	150
Digging in yard	Moderate	30 minutes	190
Dusting	Moderate	30 minutes	75
Mowing lawn	Pushing hand mower	30 minutes	200
	Pushing power mower	30 minutes	145
Raking lawn	Moderate	30 minutes	130
Sexual activity	Conventional, familiar partner	15 minutes	25
Stair climbing	Moderate, upstairs	10 minutes	100
	Moderate, downstairs	10 minutes	30
Washing car by hand	Moderate	30 minutes	100
Recreational Activities			
Aerobic dance	Moderate	30 minutes	200
Biking	Moderate	30 minutes	250
Calisthenics	Moderate	30 minutes	130
Golfing	Pulling clubs	30 minutes	145
Jogging	12 minutes/mile	30 minutes	200
Rope jumping	Moderate	15 minutes	200
Skiing	Downhill or water	30 minutes	200
	Cross-country	30 minutes	315
Swimming	Moderate	30 minutes	230
Tennis	Doubles	30 minutes	160
	Singles	30 minutes	200
Walking	Moderate	30 minutes	125
Yoga (Hatha)	Moderate	30 minutes	130

Source: The No Sweat Exercise Plan. Lose Weight, Get Healthy, and Live Longer. New York: McGraw-Hill; 2006.

OLDER and SEDENTARY

- Maintaining or increasing physical activity levels from a baseline equivalent to meeting the minimum public health recommendations has the greatest population health impact, with these trajectories being responsible for preventing nearly one in two deaths associated with physical inactivity. In addition to shifting the population towards meeting the minimum physical activity recommendations, public health efforts should also focus on the maintenance of physical activity levels, specifically preventing declines over mid to late life.
- Replacing 30 min/d of sitting time with either LPA or moderate to vigorous physical activity (MVPA) was associated with a lower risk for mortality, although this varied according to activity level.
- Even low levels of physical activity were associated with a mortality benefit compared with no physical activity among older adults. There was a minimal improvement in mortality in comparing basic compliance with physical activity guidelines with high levels of exercise.
- Replacing 30 minutes of sedentary time with either LPA or MVPA was associated with a lower risk for mortality among older adults. In particular, adults at age 75 benefited from less sedentary time, but the mortality benefit associated with reducing sedentary time did not apply to adults with high baseline levels of physical activity.
- Even mild amounts of LPA among adults promote greater longevity.
- Middle aged and older adults, including those with cardiovascular disease and cancer, stand to gain substantial longevity benefits by becoming more physically active, irrespective of past physical activity levels and established risk factors—including overall diet quality, body mass index, blood pressure, triglycerides, and cholesterol.
- At the population level, meeting and maintaining at least the minimum public health recommendations (150 minutes per week of moderate-intensity physical activity) would potentially prevent 46% of deaths associated with physical inactivity

CHAPTER 7.
EXERCISE PROGRAMS

START-UP, LOW KEY, ADVANCED and HIGH END

The following are the various researched programs. Your choice will depend on your age, physical status, available time and attitude.

> **Live Longest recommends SIT and Resistance Training on alternate days and HIPA**

SIT involves using an Exercise Bike which may be a prohibitive expense, but it takes only 40 seconds three times a week and does not damage your joints as may jogging.

Resistance Training should be done on alternate days and of one large muscle group (e.g. Upper body one day, legs next time, body next). The cheapest equipment is just socks or bags filled with sand or rubber tubes of increasing resistance of which a set can be as cheap as $10 at Aldi.

Intensity Definitions
Sitting = 0
Exhaustion = 10
Moderate = 5 to 6 with a noticeable increase in breathing and heart rate
These are *in addition* to present normal daily activities

Muscle-strengthening Activity
Minimum 2 days a week
8 to 10 exercises using major muscle groups on non-consecutive days
Weight = To allow 10 to 15 repetitions per exercise

Weight Definitions
No movement = 0
Maximum effort = 10
Moderate = 5 to 6
High Intensity = 7 to 8

Flexibility (or Joint Range of Movements)
   At least 10 minutes of flexibility activities
   Minimum   =   2 days
   Preferable   =   Every day with aerobic and strength exercises
   10 to 30 seconds of static large muscle stretching
   Repeat x 3 to 4 times

Balancing Exercises
   Most important to reduce falls.
   Someone is admitted to hospital every 8 minutes with an osteoporotic fracture – usually the result of a fall.
   50% of women and 30% of men will suffer these.
   Balance exercises are most important.

Activity Plan
A tailored personal Activity Plan should be mapped out to suit especially those over 65.

NEW CRITERIA

Previous exercise guidelines recommended at least 150 minutes of moderate exercise or 75 minutes of vigorous activity per week, ideally spread out over several days but a recent study found that even brief trips up and down stairs would count toward accumulated exercise minutes and reducing health risks so long as the intensity reaches a moderate or vigorous level. Moderate exertion was defined as brisk walking at a pace that makes it hard to carry a conversation. Boosting that pace to a jog would be vigorous exercise for most people, he said. The most dramatic improvements in the overall risk for death and disease can occur with a relatively small amount of effort, and the more you do, the better the benefits.

People who got less than 20 minutes of moderate or vigorous activity each day had the highest risk of death. Those who got 60 minutes per day cut their risk of death by more than half -- 57 percent. Getting at least 100 minutes of moderate or vigorous activity per day cut risk of death by 76 percent, the data showed

RECOMMENDATIONS (adjust for the regime you choose)

Aerobic (Endurance) activity
    HIIPA
    Moderate intensity (eg brisk walking), 30 minutes, 5 days a week
or   Vigorous intensity (eg jogging), 20 minutes, 3 days a week
or   Combinations thereof

Climbing a few flights of stairs on your lunch hour can provide a quick and effective workout. The health benefits are significant.

IF YOU ARE BREATHING HARD
YOU HAVE BEEN EXERCISING EFFICIENTLY –
MUSCLES ARE BEING TONED

PROGRESSIVE REGIMES TO SELECT FROM

From Walking To High End Exercises

More achievable and age relevant regimes are covered progressively.
Do what suits you best and can do for your age and condition…but do it.
Get mobile, get up, get going, get flexible.
Sedentary behaviour—prolonged sitting—has been shown to increase risk of higher mortality from all causes and chronic disease, particularly cancer, diabetes and cardiovascular disease.

Walking Classification: Steps / day

    i.   <5000: 'sedentary lifestyle index'
    ii. 5000–7499'low active' = typical daily activity (no sports/ exercise)
    iii. 7500–9999 'somewhat active' includes some volitional activities (and/or elevated occupational activity demands)
    iv. ≥10 000: 'active'
    v. >12 500: 'highly active' and maintain weight loss

If you want to walk short bursts of 5 minutes they accumulate to be as good as doing it all at once.
6x5 = 30 minutes a day = 150 minutes a week and as good as continuous.

Walking as few as 4400 steps per day may decrease the risk for all-cause mortality among older women, according to a study published online May 29 in *JAMA Internal Medicine*. The risk for death fell with increasing number of steps per day, and these benefits levelled off after 7500 steps/day and 8,300 steps provided protection against Alzheimer's.

PROGRAMS

1) **Minimal. Start 0 – 4 weeks**
2) **Current 'Official' WHO Guidelines**
3) **The Three Largest Recent Studies:**
4) **Harvard**
5) **James Cook**
6) **JRS**
7) **Slow and Steady Jogging**
8) **Work up a sweat: It could save your life**
9) **Fractionized Exercise**
10) **High Intensity Training (HIT)**
11) **Home Hit (HHIT)**
12) **SIT and GET FIT**
13) **SSIT Short SIT _ Recommended**
14) **High Intensity Circuit Training (HICT) Using Body Weight**

1) Minimal. Start 0 – 4 weeks

- Decrease sedentary time by two to three hours in a 12-hour day.
- Make sure you stand every 30 minutes.
- Begin gently. Push a little as you get fitter
- Work up to it! **No s**udden unusual vigorous exercise
- Body awareness - focus on balance, agility & flexibility eg Tai Chi, Yoga
- Range of Motion - warm up with a walk / hot bath then do feel good stretches
- Ease into resistance training when you've developed a base fitness
- Walking as above
- or Moving - whole body involvement: walking, water aerobics, elliptical trainer, treadmill 20 to 40 min alternate days. Increase speed, frequency and duration according to how you feel / get fit but avoid pushing too hard.
- or SSIT: Exercise bike 40 seconds x3 times / week

2) Current 'Official' WHO Guidelines

150 but preferably 300 minutes of low intensity physical activity or 75 minutes but preferably 150 minutes of vigorous physical activity weekly. Those over 65 who can't manage 150 minutes should increase lighter activities.

3) The Three Largest Recent Studies:

1. Harvard University	Premature Mortality % Reduction
No exercise	No benefit
Little but less than recommended	20%
150 min / wk moderate	31%
450 min / wk (> 1hr /day)	39% BEST
X 10 more (25 hours per week)	No further benefit
2. James Cook University	
As above but with vigorous bursts	
30% Vigorous	Further 9%
> 30%	Further 13%
3. 10-20-30 JRS Interval Program	Improved times, lower BP and other health markers

i. Harvard
450 minutes of activity per week of which 30 minutes should be vigorous = 39% less likely to die prematurely

ii. James Cook
The study by James Cook University, also showed there was a dose-response relationship between moderate to vigorous physical activity and mortality. In this study the risk of all-cause mortality was reduced 34% among those who reported exercising moderately (such as gentle swimming, social tennis, or household chores) or vigorously (such as jogging, aerobics or competitive tennis) for 10 to 149 minutes per week. For those who exercised 150 to 299 and 300 minutes or more per week, all-cause mortality was reduced 47% and 54%, respectively i.e. a slightly larger reduction in all-cause mortality in men and women who did more vigorous physical activity. The risk of mortality for those who included some vigorous activity was 9 to 13 per cent lower, compared with those who only undertook moderate activity. The research indicated that even small amounts of vigorous activity could help reduce the risk of early death

iii. The JRS (Jog, Run Sprint) 10-20-30 Intermittent Program
This fitness program is shorter and may be of equal benefit:
    a. More pleasant than other longer or more strenuous programs
    b. Less drop-out rates
    c. Suitable for nonexperienced to elite athletes
    d. Same or better results than longer programs
    e. Improved endurance performances (times)
    f. No equipment necessary, no heart rate monitor
    g. No gym membership
    h. Solo or groups
    i. Improved social interaction with groups
    j. Great with your dog(s)
    k. Most easily adhered to: 10 seconds Vs 4 minutes
    l. Lowers blood pressure

The study examined the effect of training by the 10-20-30 concept on performance, blood pressure (BP), and skeletal muscle angiogenesis (blood vessel growth) as well as the feasibility of completing high-intensity interval training in local running communities. One hundred sixty recreational runners were divided into either a control group or a 10-20-30 training group replacing two of three weekly training sessions with 10-20-30 training for 8 weeks and performance of a 5-km run (5-K) and BP was measured. VO_{2max} was measured and resting muscle biopsies were taken in a subgroup of runners.

10-20-30 improved 5-K time (38 s) and lowered systolic BP (2 ± 1 mmHg). For hypertensive subjects BP was lowered even more by 5 ± 4 and 3 ± 2 mmHg, respectively.

10-20-30 increased VO_{2max} but did not influence muscle fiber area, distribution or capillarization, whereas the expression of the pro-angiogenic vascular endothelial growth factor (VEGF) was lowered by 22%. These results suggest that 10-20-30 training is an effective and easily implemented training intervention improving endurance performance, VO_{2max} and lowering BP in recreational runners, but does not affect muscle morphology and reduces muscle VEGF.

VO_2 max is the maximum rate of oxygen consumption as measured during incremental exercise, most typically on a motorized treadmill. It is a laboratory test and an increase indicates you are getting fitter.

Instructions:
Actually it is 30-20-10 : Jog, run, sprint.
30 seconds: Run, cycle or row gently and relaxed for 30 seconds
20 seconds: Ease into accelerating to a moderate pace for 20 seconds
10 seconds: Sprint as hard as you can for 10 seconds to cover as much distance as possible (remember the Olympic 100 meter dash is around 10 seconds!).
Repeat to a total of five sets in a row without a pause.
Rest for 2 minutes by standing or very slow walking.
Repeat the five sets once more.
Finish.
The whole session is 12 minutes (less warm up and cool down).
If and when ready or if fit, do a third set.
Rest the next day. Do not do the 10-20-30 two days in a row. You may do light exercise only but perhaps resistance exercise of your upper torso would be best.
Start by replacing one or two of your usual weekly workouts. Progress slowly.
For those over 65 who may find exercise difficult it has been recommended to reduce sedentary time and increase light activities which may prove more realistic and pave the way to more intense exercise. See later.

4) Slow and Steady Jogging
A Danish 12-year prospective study found that slow and moderate joggers live longer than both their fast-paced and sedentary peers and those who exercised strenuously had similar all-cause mortality to those who didn't jog at all. Two to three times per week was found to be the ideal frequency and the optimal pace was slow or average. The lowest mortality were those who jogged 1–2-4 hours per week- 70% lower mortality than the sedentary non-joggers.

5) Work up a sweat: It could save your life
Any amount of leisure-time physical activity is associated with a significantly lower risk of death when compared with no physical activity at all. Those who did a little still had a 20% lower mortality risk compared with individuals who did no exercise at all. In the US, the current guidelines recommend exercise each week for health benefits. Those who achieved the minimum recommended physical-activity target of 150 to 300 minutes of moderate-intensity exercise or 75 to 150 minutes of vigorous-intensity had a 31% lower risk of dying compared with the physically inactive. Those who did a lot more, such as those exceeding the weekly recommendations, had an even larger reduction in mortality risk. Compared with those who did no exercise at all, individuals who performed approximately three to five times

the recommended minimum had a near 40% reduction in the risk of dying. For moderate-intensity physical activity, the maximum benefit in terms of mortality reduction occurred at levels around the weekly recommended minimum, with little to be gained by going beyond that amount

> *Physical activity that makes you puff and sweat is key to avoiding an early death*

Best Results
The best scientific advice in 2015 was that running for 20 to 30 minutes, or about a mile-and-a-half to three miles, twice per week would appear to be optimum.

Such runners generally weighed less and had a lower risk of obesity than people who jogged fewer than five miles per week or (more commonly) not at all, and were less likely to experience high blood pressure, cholesterol problems, diabetes, strokes, certain cancers and arthritis.

Running a few additional miles each week could be worthwhile if worried about middle-aged spread, because additional mileage is generally associated with better weight control and allows one to eat more calories.

Some evidence suggested that running strenuously for more than about an hour every day could slightly increase someone's risks for heart problems, as well as for running-related injuries and disabilities.

SIT at 40 seconds would seem the same as running for 45 minutes after measuring muscle glycogen in both. Less bother, less joint damage, faster but you do need an Exercise Bike.

6) Fractionized Exercise
Three 10 minute bouts of walking beat 30 minutes
A study examined whether breaking up exercise into small, manageable segments throughout the day would are as beneficial as the same length of exercise in one continuous bout.

A group of adult volunteers who were generally healthy except for early symptoms of high blood pressure (Hypertension) which is one of the primary risk factors for heart disease and stroke. Those in the study tended to have an average daily blood pressure around an unhealthy 140/90 and a tendency and a tendency to occasional higher spikes during the day.

Many studies show that prehypertension responds well to exercise. However, these studies all employed moderate exercise sessions lasting for an uninterrupted 30 minutes or so per day. This is the common standard for improving health.

It was then examined whether dividing 30 minutes of exercise into three 10 minute sessions spaced throughout the day would have a better outcome. Volunteers walked briskly at an intensity equaling about 75% of each volunteer's maximum heart rate during three 10-minute sessions at 9:30am, 1:30pm and 5:30pm. They also completed one 30 minute session of brisk walking one afternoon on a separate day, and on the final day they did no exercise.

The result was that breaking up the daily exercise into three short sessions was significantly more effective than a single half-hour session. Average blood pressure was lowered, as well as the number of times their blood pressure spiked above 140/90.

This confirms yet again that sitting for long periods throughout the day is damaging to health and longevity, and it is highly beneficial to get up and move around. Many people think that 30 minutes of exercise each day is just too hard or takes up too much time, but now there is proof that a brisk 10 minute walk or other exercise is a great thing to do.

For blood pressure control, fractionized exercise was actually more effective than a single 30 minute bout.

This study joins a growing body of evidence suggesting that for many purposes, short, cumulative exercise sessions are remarkably beneficial.

Another study of children and teenagers found that repeated bouts of running or other physical activity lasting as little as five minutes at a time reduced their poor cholesterol profiles, wide waistlines and above-average blood pressure readings as much as longer exercise sessions did.

Other studies found that exercising sporadically throughout the day aids in weight control, particularly for older women. They also showed that short, random exercise sessions improved aerobic fitness among previously sedentary people as much as a single, longer workout did. The short sessions were also more likely to be maintained over the long term.

However, fractionized exercise has its limits. You won't be an athlete.

Any movement is good
Even if you are not exercising and getting your heart and breathing rates up, any movement is beneficial. Today's lifestyles mean sitting for long periods - working, studying, eating, travelling, watching TV, relaxing. Sitting still for an hour is damaging and dangerous - and it can be countered just by getting up and walking around.

7) High Intensity Training (HIT)
High-intensity training only for Trained Athletes
High-intensity 'sprint training' may cause damage if you have not done it. Signs of stress in the muscle tissues of non-athlete, untrained subjects after ultra-intense leg and arm cycling exercises have been found with untrained subjects then having weakened ability to fight off free radicals, molecules that can alter DNA and harm healthy cells.

NOTE: SIT, see below, does not impose such demands or risks.

High-Intensity Training No Better Than Conventional Training
High-intensity interval training and steady-state training have similar effects on aerobic and anaerobic fitness, steady-state cycling or to one of two high-intensity interval training protocols. Steady-state cycling was compared to two high-intensity interval training protocols (Meyer and Tabata). There were significant improvements on all measures of exercise capacity in all three groups. However, when all measures were combined, the differences among the three groups were not significant.

Table. Improvements in Exercise Capacity

Measure	Steady-State Protocol	Meyer Protocol	Tabata Protocol
Maximum oxygen consumption, mL/kg	19	18	18
Peak aerobic work, W/kg	17	14	24
Peak anaerobic output, W/kg	8	5	9
Average anaerobic output, W/kg	4	6	7

The Tabata protocol required less time to achieve the results, but the participants needed more time to recover from their intense exercise, potentially canceling the benefit. Ratings on the Exercise Enjoyment Scale indicated that the participants liked the exercise less and less as the study wore on. They liked the Tabata protocol least of the three, and the steady-state protocol most.

8) Home Hit (HHIT)

A study compared
1) a supervised, lab-based cycling HIT programme,
2) the Government-recommended 150 minutes of moderate intensity exercise
3) a home-based HIT programme of simple body weight exercises suitable for people with low fitness and low mobility and performed without equipment. For all of these regimens, the exercise was performed three times per week.

They found that the home-based HIT was as effective as both the Government-recommended 150 minutes and the supervised, lab-based HIT programme for improving fitness in obese individuals.

Home-HIT reduces barriers to exercise, such as time, cost, and access, and increases adherence in previously inactive individuals gives people a more attainable exercise goal.

SSIT, of course, does the same.

9) SIT and GET FIT

A single minute of very intense exercise produces health benefits similar to longer, traditional endurance training.

Sprint Interval Training (SIT) was compared using Key health indicators including cardiorespiratory fitness and insulin sensitivity, a measure of how the body regulates blood sugar, to moderate-intensity continuous training (MICT) as recommended in public health guidelines.

The SIT protocol workout totaled just 10 minutes, including a 2-minute warm-up, three 20-second 'all-out' cycle sprints, 3-minute cool down and two minutes of easy cycling for recovery between the hard sprints.

The study compared the SIT protocol with a group who performed 45 minutes of continuous cycling at a moderate pace, plus the same warm-up and cool down. After 12 weeks of training, the results were remarkably similar, even though the MICT protocol involved five times as much exercise and a five-fold greater time commitment.

10) SSIT (Short SIT)

> A later study found that two 20 second bursts of intense SIT exercise bike pedaling depleted muscle glycogen as much as a 45 minute run did. Live Longest recommends this exercise, three times a week on alternate days with weight training on alternate days.

11) High Intensity Circuit Training (HICT) Using Body Weight

Circuit Training – different exercises at different sites for different body areas – invented at Leeds University in 1953 - combines both aerobic and resistance training. It offers 'Maximum Results with Minimal Investment' as it can be done using one's own body weight no special equipment is needed, can be done anywhere, anytime (good for travellers). A series of 12 exercises ensures that all large muscle groups are exercised in an order allowing opposing muscle groups to alternate between working and resting. The High Intensity trade-off for its short duration and lack of any special equipment is that the participant must be able to handle a great degree of discomfort for a relatively short duration. As such it is probably restricted to those who are already somewhat fit and not the obese or those with any medical conditions.

SUMMARY:
- Running 20 to 30 minutes, or about a mile-and-a-half to three miles, twice per week would now appear to be optimum as to practicality
- 450 minutes of activity per week of which 30 minutes should be vigorous = 39% less likely to die prematurely
- 150 minutes moderate physical activity / exercise a week = 31% less likely to die prematurely
- 10-20-30 secs mild, moderate intense exercise x 5 on alternate days = Same benefits

But
Live Longest recommends SSIT (Exercise Bike) + HIPA

- **Two 20 secs bursts three times a week is the equivalent of running 45 mins. Sitting down – no joint damage**
- **HIPA: Optimising and maximising normal activities**

And alternating days: Light weights, socks, sand-bags or rubber tubes/ bands

SUGGESTED EXERCISES FOR ALL AGE GROUPS

All Ages

Brisk walking for only 20 minutes a day burns about 700 calories a week, results in a 30 to 40 percent reduced risk of coronary heart disease and can be performed even by the elderly.

Regular physical activity also should include resistance exercise such as lifting weights, which can even be safely performed in the elderly and in patients with heart failure. The general health benefits of resistance training for middle-aged and older adults are many, including the prevention or limitation of age-related sarcopenia, improved maintenance of muscle mass strength, and a decreased risk of osteoporosis-related bone fractures, falls, physical disability, and mortality.

Tennis players live longest. Is it the arm swinging that drives our upper body and brain circulation to maximise efficiency.

Our bodies biologically start to decline aged 35 along with cardiovascular fitness.

Weight -Resistance Training cane be with sand filled socks, elastic bands but also every-day trying to increase lifting shopping or whatever.

20s

Maximise running while you can: Sprinting, tennis, running team sports also rowing, cycling, swimming and circuits.

The 20s represents your physical prime. Optimise it by building strength and muscle.

Recommend 30 minutes of moderate physical activity most days of the week, including strength endurance classes, such as circuits, and cardio-vascular activities i.e. Weights and running.

30s

Sedentary job, marriage and kids reduce available time and activity. Allocate "Me Time". Consider joining a sports club (high intensity tennis, jogging) or a gym with a commitment you can keep.

Try 25-minute run in your lunch hour.

Childbirth: Pelvic floor exercises with planks, side planks, bridging, pilates and yoga.

Muscle naturally starts to decline. Leave longer recovery times.

40s

The dreaded middle-aged spread and increasing stress and increasingly hectic lifestyles can get in the way of exercise with increasing risk of type-2 diabetes and high cholesterol.

Try brisk walking, spin classes, jogging and swimming.

Try and find the time for endurance activities such as long-distance cycling and running but such running has long-term hip and knee problems. Swimming is arguably the best exercise.

Weights and impact (fast walking, jogging) are however, beneficial to prevent osteoporosis,

Heavy weights and high intensity interval training three times a week is to be recommended.

Core development work is important now to prevent back problems: Try pilates.

50s

To keep up muscle mass and heart health try cardio activity such as walking and swimming three times a week with weighs, dead lifts, bench chest presses, push-ups and squats on alternate days. One USA 58-year-old says does 400 squats a week.

Don't slow down or you'll end up in a nursing home.

Yoga maintains and improves flexibility and pilates strengthens your core. It is sad to see old people unable to bend to put their socks on or clip their nails. Get flexible!

Do Balance Exercises. Stimulate mobility and co-ordination with throwing, catching or hitting, Golf, tennis, or bag boxing.

60s

Get your doctor's advice. See Book 3 for potential cardio-vascular problems.

Concentrate on flexibility, mobility and coordination / balance.

Moderate intensity cardiovascular work, such as jogging, power walking, gardening, dancing or swimming a few times a week is important. But you also need to do some interval training to condition the heart and lungs. That could be walking fast up a relatively steep hill for 45 seconds and strolling back down, repeating 6-8 times.

We recommend SIT or SSIT.

Dancing is arguably the best total workout. Get jiving!

70s and beyond

If tennis is difficult as costs and distances increase as partners decrease, consider table tennis – it's a great workout. Dancing, again, is great. Swimming marvellous.

Back pain is more common and core exercises needed (ask your physio about "Multifidus exercises – to be crude this in effect means tightening your anus to try and make it reach your belly button).

Maintain or increase flexibility. Hatha yoga is to be recommended.

Home: The 12-minute exercise plan devised for the Royal Canadian Air Force in the 70s (?).

Standing up from a chair, standing knee bends and marching on the spot, for five, one-minute exercises to be done twice a day for 65- to 80-year-olds, resulted, after four weeks, in a 2% increase in quad size (the gold standard for muscle growth) and a 5 to 6% increase in strength in people had never exercised before.

Authors Note: Dancing, table tennis, yoga: I am intrigued by my oldest patients late 80s and early 90s who either dance or play table tennis.

Tai Chi

- Several health benefits for those over 65 years
- Better posture, balance, flexibility
- Alleviate joint pain (Osteo and Rheumatoid Arthritis)
- In 10 weeks maintain balance, strength, reduce sway and increase walking speed resulting in 47.5% less falls
- In 15 weeks 15min x2 /day improved Cardio Respiratory System

  i.e. improved physical and psychological measures

Interval Training For 'Belly Fat' in 70-year-olds

Aging leads to a gradual decrease in lean body mass (LBM). LBM is the entire weight of your body minus the weight associated with fat tissue. As we age, fat distribution in the body can shift, and often increases in the belly region. This is a health concern for older adults, because so-called "belly fat" (also known as "central obesity") is associated with a greater risk for heart disease than general obesity.

A 10-week, easy-to-perform, personalized, progressive vigorous-intensity interval training among 70-year-olds with "belly fat" study was published in the *Journal of the American Geriatrics Society*.

The program consisted of short, supervised training sessions, performed in a group setting, three times per week for 10 weeks and taught to perform body-weight-training exercises with minimal use of equipment, at first for 18 minutes, alternating exercise with rest periods in a ratio of 40/20 (for example, 40 seconds of work and then 20 seconds of rest). The participants worked up to a 36-minute training period as their training volume gradually increased.

Participants in the exercise group decreased their fat mass by nearly two pounds and gained about one pound of lean body weight compared to the control group.

The researchers concluded that 10 weeks of vigorous intensity interval training improved body composition in older adults with belly fat. Those in the exercise group saw a nearly tripled decrease in their total fat mass compared with participants in the control group. The exercise group also saw positive effects on total lean body mass. The "do-ability" of the exercise program was reflected in the high attendance rates (89 percent) for the training sessions.

CHAPTER 8.
OVER 65s

A tailored personal Activity Plan should be mapped out to suit especially those over 65.

The older one becomes the more difficult the exercises and the need to modify them. Moderate and vigorous exercise targets may not be achievable. But, given the dose-response benefits for physical activity and health benefits, continued exercise is vital so increase light activities but most importantly, reducing sedentary time is where to start.

Light exercise is more appealing to people over 65 and such activities do not generally require medical clearance. Older adults who participated in light intensity exercise activities for 300 minutes or more were 18 percent healthier, overall, than peers who did not do as much. They had lower body mass index (BMI), smaller waist circumference, better insulin rates and were less likely to have chronic diseases.

Current medical recommendations suggest that all adults engage in 150 minutes of moderate exercise each week but exercise of less intensity, done more often, produced similar health benefits.

Guidance
- "Low-dose" moderate-to-vigorous physical activity of, say, 75 minutes per week or 15 minutes per day, such as brisk walking, cycling, swimming or gymnastics and possibly associated with leisure time physical activity or daily life activities for five days a week would be a suitable first target for the elderly and significantly reduced mortality by 22%.
- Any reduction, however, even in low levels of activity, exposed the elderly to a higher risk of death.
- In the general population 30 minutes at least five days a week (or 150 minutes per week) has been shown to reduce the average risk of death by 30%.
- 30 mins of at least moderate intensity physical activity on at least 5 days a week will improve health
- Two 15 min periods of moderate activity in a day can be beneficial & a good way to start
- Every little bit counts toward the 30 mins total. Do little and often to start
- Maximum benefit gained with 20 mins of vigorous endurance activity three time a week, 20 mins of strengthening activity twice a week, plus daily stretching, balance and coordination activities

- Any activity is better than none - even once a week
- It's never too late to start
- Benefits only remain as long as you exercise
- Again Live Longest recommends SSIT and HIPA as the fastest, gentlest and easiest

Participating in a walking group may dramatically improve overall health. Participants of group walking showed significant reduction in mean differences for systolic blood pressure, resting heart rate, body fat, body mass index (BMI), and total cholesterol.
The suggested target for older adults (≥ 65) is the same as for other adults (18-64): 60 to 150 minutes a week of slow-moderate intensity activity which can be in bouts of 10 minutes or more.

It is often expressed as 30 minutes of brisk walking or equivalent activity two to three days a week. Physical activity to improve strength should also be done at least two days a week.

While the 150 minute target is widely disseminated to health professionals and the public, many people, especially in older age groups, find it hard to achieve this level of activity.

It is suggested to increase their level of activity by small amounts rather than focus on the recommended levels.

The suggested target for older adults (≥ 65) is the same as for other adults (18-64): 150 minutes a week of moderate intensity activity in bouts of 10 minutes or more. It is often expressed as 30 minutes of brisk walking or equivalent activity five days a week, although 75 minutes of vigorous intensity activity spread across the week, or a combination of moderate and vigorous activity are sometimes suggested. Physical activity to improve strength should also be done at least two days a week.

The 150 minute target is widely disseminated to health professionals and the public. However, many people, especially in older age groups, find it hard to achieve this level of activity.

The 150 minute target, although warranted, may overshadow other less concrete elements of guidelines. These include finding ways to do more lower intensity lifestyle activity. As people get older, activity may become more relevant for sustaining the strength, flexibility, and balance required for independent living in addition to the strong associations with hypertension, coronary heart disease, stroke, diabetes, breast cancer, and colon cancer. Observational data have confirmed associations between increased physical activity and reduction in musculoskeletal conditions such as arthritis, osteoporosis, and sarcopenia, and better cognitive acuity and mental health. Although these links may be modest and some lack evidence of causality, they may provide sufficient incentives for many people to be more active.

Older people should increase their level of activity by small amounts rather than focus on the recommended levels.

One again, Live Longest is impressed and recommends SSIT: Two 20 second bursts on an exercise bicycle. This allows sitting down, no pounding of knee or hip joints and the 20 second "bursts" can be started gently and slowly and increased slowly. A bike with push-pull handlebars also exercises the upper body-arms.

It is to be emphasised that intense exercise doesn't eliminate the hazard of intense sitting. Sedentary behavior was defined as "waking behaviors characterized by little physical movement and low-energy expenditure," including watching television and sitting. Increased sedentary time was associated with significant, independent increases in risk for all-cause, cardiovascular, and cancer mortality, as well as cardiovascular disease, cancer, and type 2 diabetes incidence. Increased exercise blunted — but did not completely eliminate — the excess risks associated with sedentary behavior.

The potential of high intensity interval training in managing the same chronic diseases, as well as reducing indices of cardio-metabolic risk in healthy adults, has emerged. This vigorous training typically comprises multiple 3-4 minute bouts of high intensity exercise interspersed with several minutes of low intensity recovery, three times a week. Live Longest recommends SSIT which SSIT is shorter.

Staying active, even later in life, can help reduce muscle loss.
Exercise is an important contributor to functional performance from which even non-athletes can benefit. Elderly people who were elite athletes in their youth or later in life who still compete as Masters Athletes have much healthier muscles at the cellular level compared to those of non-athletes. Their legs were 25 per cent stronger on average and had about 14 per cent more total muscle mass. With normal aging, the nervous system lose motor neurons, leading to a loss of motor units, reduced muscle mass, less strength, speed and power. That process speeds up substantially past age 60.

Age Decline in Activity
Moderate and vigorous physical activity decrease across all ages and the decline in higher intensity activities with increasing age. Only in the youngest adult age group is the average level above 30 minutes a day. The proportions of time spent sedentary rises with age from 55% (7.7 hours) at 20-29 years to 67% (9.6 hours) in those aged 70-79 years. As so little time is spent in moderate and vigorous activities, higher sedentary time in older adults reflects less time spent in light activity.

Chase That Ball when 63-75
Long-term recreational soccer training produced a number of marked improvements in health profile for 63-75 year old untrained men -- including a reduced risk of developing cardiovascular diseases and diabetes. After 4 months' soccer training, the cardiovascular fitness scores improved by 15%, interval work capacity increased by 43% and functional capacity by 30%. After a year there was a 3% reduction in BMI purely from the loss of fat mass, with an increased ability to control blood sugar and an improved capacity to handle harmful oxygen radicals, which could otherwise cause increased oxidative stress in the body and have a harmful effect on many vital cell functions.

Physical Activity and Risk of Coronary Heart Disease and Stroke in Older Adults
With advancing age the ability to perform some types of Physical Activity (PA) might decrease, making light-moderate exercise such as walking especially important to meet recommendations. Greater PA was inversely associated with coronary heart disease, stroke (especially ischemic stroke), and total CVD, even in those ≥75 years. Walking pace, distance, and overall walking score, leisure-time activity, and exercise intensity were each associated with lower risk. For example, in comparison with a walking pace <2 mph, those that habitually walked at a pace >3 mph had a lower risk of coronary heart disease, stroke and CVD. This data provides empirical evidence supporting PA. In particular, walking, to reduce the incidence of CVD among older adults especially in those >75 years.

Weekend warriors
Weekend cramming does offer some benefits too
Healthy men who burnt off 1000 Cal in one or two weekly bursts are 60% less likely to die over a 10 year period than sedentary men who expended <500 Cal.

Exercise and the Brain

The frontal and pre-frontal areas of the brain, which mediate executive processes – *inhibition, selection, planning, coordination of perception, working memory and action* – are especially at risk for age-related decline. In contrast, other areas of the brain, such as the occipital lobe and motor cortex, which underlie visual and motor processes are relatively immune to the ageing process. Preservation of this executive functioning should therefore be our main priority.

A physically active lifestyle seems to maintain and enhance specific aspects of cognitive function in older men and women and the benefits seem to increase with more vigorous activity participation.

CHAPTER 9.
SOME AGE CHANGES = EXERCISE DEFICIENCY

Sarcopaenia: is the loss of muscle mass and strength or atrophy with age

> Increases after 30
> Even healthy people lose strength @ 1 - 2% pa and power @ 3 - 4%pa
> After age 20   =   2 – 3 % pa
> After age 65   =   10% pa
> 65 – 70 yrs   =   13 to 24% pa
> After 80   =   50%
> i.e. there is a loss of some 35% to 40% of muscle between ages 20 to 80 years

* 30 yr olds need only 50 - 60% quadriceps to rise from sitting
* 90 yr olds need 95% and hence we see the elderly now struggling to rise from low chairs
* Most rapid loss for men is between 40 and 60 years and for women after 60.
* Fat increases when muscle mass decreases
* In the English National Fitness Survey nearly half the women & 15% of men aged 70 – 74 were too weak to be confident of being able to mount a 30 cm step without a handrail
* It's never too late as per studies on 55 to 75 yr olds
* Muscle atrophy is due to a gradual and selective loss of fast-twitch type ii muscle fibres which are then replaced by fat and connective tissue which reduces velocity and strength
* Maximum Oxygen Uptake Rate (VO2 max) defines capacity for endurance exercise
* A decrease in muscle mass decreases the VO2 max at the rate of 1% per annum
* This is reflected in a decreased aerobic capacity
* Resistance training increases the VO2 max
* Often overlooked is the value of strength-building exercises. Once you reach your 50s and beyond, strength (or resistance) training is critical to preserving the ability to perform the most ordinary activities of daily living — and to maintain an active and independent lifestyle.

The average 30-year-old will lose about a quarter of his or her muscle strength by age 70 and half of it by age 90   or 1% of bone mass per year after age 40 due to inadequate muscle exercise. This then leads to osteoporosis. Just doing aerobic exercise is not adequate. Unless you are doing strength training, you will become weaker and less functional.

Lifetime Fitness and Musculo-Skeletal Health
Being physically active may significantly improve musculoskeletal and overall health and minimize or delay the effects of aging. An increasing amount of evidence demonstrates that we can modulate age-related decline in the musculoskeletal system. A lot of the deterioration with aging can be attributed to a more sedentary lifestyle instead of aging itself. Being physically active may significantly improve musculoskeletal and overall health, and minimize or delay the effects of aging, according to research on senior athletes (ages 65 and up). Individual progressive resistance, endurance and flexibility-balance exercise regimes are recommended.

Essential
In August 2007 the American Heart Association and the American College of Sports Medicine released a most significant joint statement targeting older adults *'Regular physical activity and muscle strengthening activity is essential for healthy ageing (which) can reduce the risk of chronic disease, premature mortality, functional limitations and disability'.*
Older adults find it difficult to meet moderate and vigorous exercise targets. Given that a dose-response exists for physical activity and health benefits a change in message to reduce sedentary time and increase light activities may prove more realistic and pave the way to more intense exercise Over the past decade, research has increased our understanding of the effects of physical activity at opposite ends of the spectrum. Sedentary behavior—too much sitting—has been shown to increase risk of chronic disease, particularly diabetes and cardiovascular disease.

Maintaining Aerobic Fitness in Middle Age Can Delay Biological Ageing by 12 Years
Aerobic exercise, such as jogging, improves the body's oxygen consumption and its metabolism but maximal aerobic power starts to fall steadily from middle age, decreasing by around 5 ml/kg/min every decade. When it falls below around 18 ml in men and 15 ml in women, it becomes difficult to do very much at all without severe fatigue.
In a typical sedentary man, the maximal aerobic power will have fallen to around 25 mil/kg/min by the age of 60, almost half of what it was at the age of 20. But evidence shows that regular aerobic exercise can slow or reverse the inexorable decline, even in later life.

Relatively high intensity aerobic exercise over a relatively long period boosted maximal aerobic power by 25%, equivalent to a gain of 6 ml/kg/min, or 10 to 12 biological years. The conservation of maximal oxygen intake increases the likelihood that the healthy elderly person will retain functional independence.

The other positive spin-offs of aerobic exercise are reduced risks of serious disease, faster recovery after injury or illness, and reduced risks of falls because of the maintenance of muscle power, balance, and coordination.

Age Weight Gain
There is both an absolute gain in weight and also a relative percentage increase in fat between 40 and 50 years from 28% to 35% with central adiposity. Thereafter it is more stable.

CHAPTER 10.
HEALTH BENEFITS

Some parts of this may seem turgid and complex but skim through it: It is devastating and if this doesn't get you off your backside then, as they say in the classics, "cop it sweet".

Fitness & Reduced Death from ALL causes

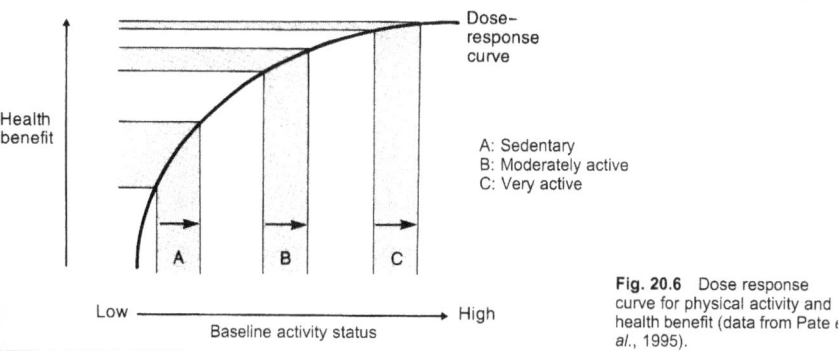

Fig. 20.6 Dose response curve for physical activity and health benefit (data from Pate et al., 1995).

This shows that as activity increases so do the benefits to our health increase proportionally.

However, as we age any movement is beneficial and can be broken into "fractionated" separate sessions as detailed.
* Intensive exercise improves the endothelium in coronary arteries i.e. it 'smoothes' the blood vessel linings
* This allows better dilation and greater blood flow

More Physical Activity Associated with Greater Reductions in Incident Disease
Higher levels of physical activity than what is recommended by the World Health Organization are associated with lower risks for five diseases, according to a meta-analysis in *The BMJ*. Most benefits appeared to occur at 3000–4000 MET minutes per week; gains beyond that level of activity were minimal.

To achieve 3000 MET minutes/week, a person could climb stairs for 10 minutes, vacuum for 15, garden for 20, run for 20, and walk or bicycle for 25 minutes every day.

Researchers analyzed 174 studies that examined disease incidence and total physical activity, including leisure time, occupation, active transportation, and domestic activity.

Compared with people who got less than the WHO's recommendation of 600 MET minutes/week, even low activity (600–3999 MET minutes/week) was associated with significant risk reduction, but the greatest risk reductions came in the high activity group (8000 MET minutes/week or more).

High activity was associated with the following relative risk reductions:
        Diabetes: 28% lower risk
        Ischemic stroke: 26%
        Ischemic heart disease: 25%
        Colon cancer: 21%
        Breast cancer: 14%

In a study of older women published 2018 in the *Journal of the American Geriatrics Society*, with each 30-minute chunk of light activities people lowered their risk of dying early by 12% compared to their more sedentary peers. And a 2018 study found that among older men, each additional half hour of light physical activity, such as walking or gardening, slashed their risk of early death by 17%.

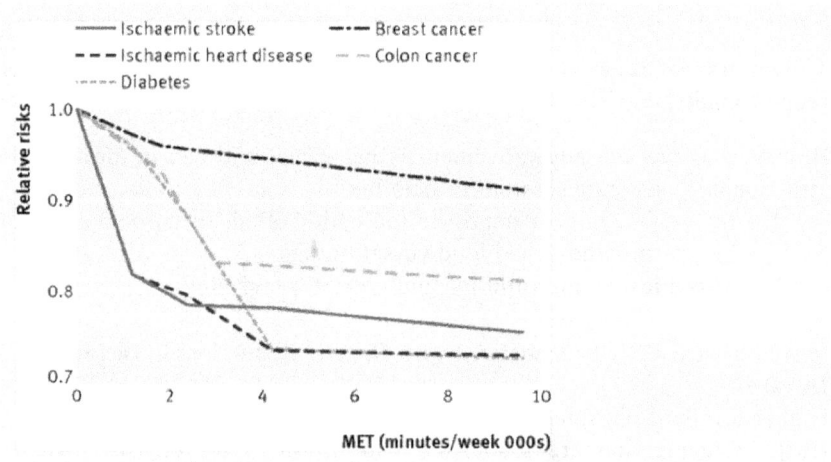

Fig 7 Continuous risk curves for association between physical activity and breast cancer, colon cancer, diabetes, ischemic heart disease, and ischemic stroke

The conclusion is that total physical activity needs to be several times higher than the current recommended minimum level of 600 MET minutes/week to optimise benefits.

To Work Out Your MET level and relevance to Death Rate

Predicted exercise capacity women	=	14.7 minus (0.13 x age)
eg 50 year old	=	14.7 – (0.13 x 50 = 6.5)
14.7 – 6.5	=	8.2 METs = 100%
85%	=	6.97
Predicted exercise capacity for men	=	14.7 minus (0.11 x age)
eg 50 year old man	=	14.7 – (0.11 x 50 = 5.5)
14.7 – 5.5	=	9.2 METs = 100%
85%	=	7.82

Exercise machines can automatically calculate METS
<85% of this predicted value doubles the death rate

Survival of the fittest

The more intense the activity the better the benefit -
There is virtually a linear reduction
Each increase of 1 MET in exercise capacity conferred a 12% improvement in survival
The relative risk of survival was four times worse for those least fit compared to those exercising most
Greater fitness results in longer survival (all causes)
Less fit people can improve survival if fitness improves
A program of regular exercise can improve fitness by 15 to 30% within 3 to 6

Exercise / week		Reduction CHD Risk
Running 1 hr (6mph)	=	42%
Wt training 30 min	=	32%
Rowing 1 hr / wk	=	18%
Brisk walking	=	18%
Low intensity walking	=	no benefit

Moderate and high physical activity led to a 1.3 and 3.7 years more in total life expectancy cf those who were sedentary (Note: Ageing is not slowed but life span increases)

- A graded program of regular exercise can improve fitness by 15 to 30 % in 3 to 6 months

- Women aged 75 to 93 years increased their strength by 24 to 30% with just 12 weeks strength training (equivalent to a 'rejuvenation' of strength by 15 -20 years)

- Women aged 80 - 93 years produced a 15% mean increase in their aerobic power to weight ratio with 24 weeks of endurance training (equivalent to a 'rejuvenation' of endurance of 15 years)

- The Women's Health Initiative Observational Study of 73,743 postmenopausal women found that both walking and vigorous exercise are associated with substantial reductions in the incidence of cardiovascular events irrespective of ethnicity, age or BMI and that prolonged sitting predicts increased cardiovascular risk.
- Women aged 50 - 79 yrs who engaged in 1.25 to 2.5 hrs of brisk walking or the equivalent had an 18% lower risk of breast cancer
- A cohort of 44,452 US men enrolled in the Health Professionals' Follow-up Study were followed from 1986 through to 1998 and the conclusions were that total physical activity and its intensity (running, rowing, weight training and walking) were each associated with reduced CVS risk.

Fit & Not Fat
In 2015, as a further example of this new preventive evidence, one of the most extensive studies ever undertaken was published: 334,161 European men and women were followed for some 12.4 years, which, apparently, corresponded to over four million person-years. By any standards this was a study of great worth and significance as, of course, were their findings. It called upon leading Universities such as Cambridge and its equivalent Universities of Europe to analyse the connection, if any, between physical activity and all-cause mortality for abdominal obesity or, in layman's terms, if being fat and sedentary led to premature death and if being active, and by what amount, allowed us live longer and of course, their conclusions provided the best recommendations possible to date.

Compared with people 'Fit - Not Fat' taken as 0% reference, the risk of death is

Fit – Not Fat	Women	Men	Risk of Death 0%
Fit – Fat	32%	25%	Higher x 25 – 32%
Unfit – Not Fat	30%	44%	Higher x 30 – 44%
Unfit - Fat	57%	49%	Higher x 59 – 57%

Compression of Morbidity. Exercise plummets with age.
As can be seen in Book 3 Successful Aging, the main aim is to compress or shorten any years of illness or disability, which invariably accompany our final years. At present we spend as much as our last 20 years with such impositions.

Keeping fit and mobile is a major contributor to Successful Ageing and Compression of Morbidity. It can be seen, however, how our exercise plummets before we even reach 30.

The message: Keep playing sport, keep physically active if you want to age well.

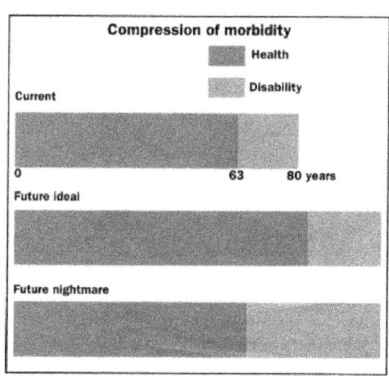
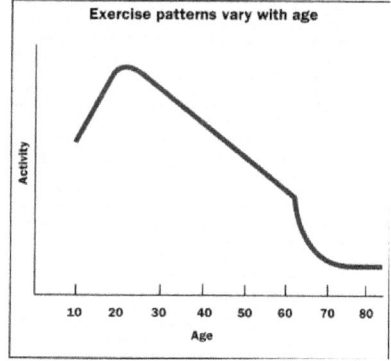

Benefits of Physical Activity

Reduced	Increased
All causes of death 30%	CVS - slowing of arterial ageing
Osteoporosis	Post Infarct survival
Insomnia	Mobility
Stress ~ Depression	Wellbeing
Fat	Fitness
CAD	Disease prevention
Strokes/ cerebral haemorrhage	Balance
Diabetes 2	Health awareness
Osteoarthritis	Cognition. Lower dementia risk.
Lipids/cholesterol	Functional status
BP	Independence
Colon cancer	Social integration
Breast Ca-postmenopausal	Quality Of Life, Mood
Ovarian cancer	Disability free years
Gallstones	Total Life Expectancy
Constipation	Better sleep (not vigorous)
COPD	Better work efficiency (12.5%)
Chronic Fatigue Syndrome	Better sex (30% less ED. >female response)
Falls/ injuries	success to quit smoking doubles
	HDL cholesterol (good)

Risk of death lowers during as people exercise more.
EuroPRevent 2016 meeting.
Compared to those who were inactive, older adults with low, medium and high activity levels had a 22 per cent, 28 per cent and 35 per cent lower risk of death, respectively.
Moderate exercise is working hard enough to raise the heart rate and breaking into a sweat. Moderate exercisers will be able to talk but not sing the words to a song.
The more physical activity older adults do, the greater the health benefit. The biggest jump in benefit was achieved at the low level of exercise, with the medium and high levels bringing smaller increments of benefit. The low level of activity, which equates to a 15 minute brisk walk each day, which is half the recommended amount, was associated with a reduced risk of death in older adults compared with those who were inactive.

> **15 Minutes A Day Keeps The Undertaker At Bay**

Even Later-Life Exercise Reduces Mortality
Regular exercise reduces the risk of death even when started in middle age, according to a study that measured the link between mortality and leisure time physical activity (LTPA). The results also show an association between LTPA and cause-specific mortality for the two leading causes of death, cardiovascular disease (CVD) and cancer and that being inactive across early adulthood but increasing LTPA later at 40 to 61 years was associated with 16% to 43% risk reduction in mortality. These mortality benefits were comparable to those associated with maintaining LTPA in all age groups from adolescence and into adulthood.

Ages 40 to 79
Middle aged and older adults, including those with cardiovascular disease and cancer, stand to gain substantial longevity benefits by becoming more physically active, irrespective of past physical activity levels and established risk factors—including overall diet quality, body mass index, blood pressure, triglycerides, and cholesterol. Maintaining or increasing physical activity levels from a baseline equivalent to meeting the minimum public health recommendations has the greatest population health impact, with these trajectories being responsible for preventing nearly one in two deaths associated with physical inactivity. In addition to shifting the population towards meeting the minimum physical activity recommendations, public health efforts should also focus on the maintenance of physical activity levels, specifically preventing declines over mid to late life.

Exercise - Physical Activity, Function, and Longevity Among the Very Old
A significant survival benefit was associated with initiating Physical Activity (PA) between ages 70 and 78 years and ages 78 and 85 years. Participation in higher levels of PA, compared with being sedentary, did not show a dose-dependent association with mortality. The PA level at age 78 was associated with remaining independent while performing activities of daily living at age 85.

AGE	8 YEAR MORTALITY %	
	PHYSICALLY ACTIVE	SEDENTARY
70	15.2	27.2
78	26.1	40.8
	3 YEAR MORTALITY %	
85	6.8	24.4

Note: This table is repeated in Successful Aging Book 3 for both convenience and emphasis

Start Young
Aerobic fitness in adolescent males is associated with reduced risk for early death — but with no protective effect seen at BMIs of 35 or greater. Furthermore, the risk of early death was higher in fit obese individuals than in unfit normal-weight individuals.

Cholesterol and Exercise
Regular aerobic exercise modestly increases HDL level. There appears to exist a minimum exercise volume for a significant increase in HDL level. Exercise duration per session was the most important element of an exercise prescription. Exercise was more effective in subjects with initially high total cholesterol levels or low body mass index.
The minimum amount of weekly exercise that appeared necessary to increase an HDL level was estimated to be 900 kcal of energy expenditure a week or 120 minutes of exercise a week.
In contrast, there was no significant association between exercise frequency or intensity.
This suggests that increasing time per session is better than doing multiple brief exercise sessions when time for exercise is limited, as is the case for many people.

To lower cholesterol
Fast walking 5+ days a week
Best Plan: Aim for 3 hrs a week
   Lipoprotein(LDL:HDL) improvement
   There is a graded response to exercise
   Low amts of moderate or high intensity exercise (walking or jogging 12 m / wk) some benefit
   High levels of high intensity - jogging 20 miles a week produces greater changes and increased (good) HDL lipoprotein cholesterol levels
   And if you don't reach the recommended levels but your regimen takes a lot of puff it's good enough to reduce CVS risk
   But if SSIT is the equivalent of a 45 minute run it would seem it should also be beneficial to both LDL and HDL

Cognitive Function
The dose – response relationship between aerobic exercise and cognition.
A clear dose-response relationship exists between exercise and cardiovascular fitness and cardiorespiratory *fitness* response was a better predictor of cognitive gains than exercise duration. Cardiovascular fitness may be the therapeutic target for achieving cognitive benefits.
Underactive or sedentary participants without cognitive impairment were randomly assigned into one of four groups: 1. no-change controls and 2. 75, 3. 150, and 4. 225 minutes/week of moderate-intensity aerobic exercise for 26 weeks.
Cognitive outcomes were derived from a battery of 16 cognitive tests assaying verbal memory, visuospatial processing, simple attention, set-shifting, and reasoning. Secondary outcomes were cardiorespiratory fitness, measured as peak oxygen consumption, and measures of functional health. The results showed that cardiorespiratory fitness increased and perceived disability decreased in a dose-dependent manner across the four groups. When analysis was restricted to those who were most adherent to the protocol, simple attention improved equivalently across all exercise groups compared with controls, and a dose-response relationship was present for visuospatial processing.
The frontal and pre-frontal areas of the brain, which mediate executive processes – *inhibition, selection, planning, coordination of perception, working memory and action* – are especially at risk for age-related decline. In contrast, other areas of the brain, such as the occipital lobe and motor cortex, which underlie visual and motor processes are relatively immune to the ageing process. Preservation of this executive functioning should therefore be our main priority.

In 1996 the Surgeon General of the USA advised that moderate, accumulated physical activity benefited cognitive function as well as physical health.

In 2007 the American College of Sports Medicine conducted a trial to determine whether physical activity was specifically and positively associated with executive function in older individuals and concluded that a physically active lifestyle is uniquely associated with specific cognitive benefits in older men and women. A physically active lifestyle seems to maintain and enhance specific aspects of cognitive function in older men and women and the benefits seem to increase with more vigorous activity participation.

Physical activity linked to greater mental flexibility in older adults
Physically fit people tend to have larger brain volumes and more intact white matter than their less-fit peers. Older adults who regularly engage in moderate to vigorous physical activity have more variable brain activity at rest than those who don't. This variability is associated with better cognitive performance. As well as accelerometers, functional MRIs were used to observe how blood oxygen levels changed in the brain over time, reflecting each participant's brain activity at rest and found spontaneous brain activity showed more moment-to-moment fluctuations in the more-active adults.

A magnetic resonance imaging study showing that greater cardiorespiratory fitness in middle aged adults is associated with more brain volume and greater white matter integrity measured five years later.

Resistance Exercise Program for Improving Cognitive Function in Elderly
6 Resistance exercises:
   1. chest press
   2. leg press
   3. vertical traction
   4. abdominal crunch
   5. leg curl
   6. lower back

Once weekly for 1 hour at 50% to 80% of 1 Maximum Repetition (RM). Maximum Repetetion - RM was found by testing on 6 apparatuses with 8 repetitions with increasing load until the maximum was obtained in 1 repetition. Cognition improvement was equal at 50% to 80% but the 80% group had a greater increase in lean mass.

Key messages
> Health and functional benefits begin with any increase above lowest levels of activity; any activity is better than none
> New guidelines now advise interspersing prolonged sitting with short bouts of standing and light activity
> Small increases in moderate activity may enable older patients to get closer to the recommended 150 minutes a week

Move more and sit less

The new USA physical-activity guidelines were updated in 2018 for the first time since 2008, and they still urge adults to do 75 minutes of vigorous (or 150 minutes of moderate) aerobic activity each week, plus muscle-strengthening sessions like weight-lifting or yoga twice a week.

Older women lowered their risk of dying early by 12% compared to their more sedentary peers with each 30-minute chunk of light activities. Older men, each additional half hour of light physical activity, such as walking or gardening, slashed their risk of early death by 17%.

A study of over 334,000 European men and women found that twice as many deaths may be attributable to lack of physical activity compared with the number of deaths attributable to obesity, and just a modest increase in physical activity could have significant health benefits.

Prolonged sitting:

There is now a clear need to reduce prolonged sitting. It is associated with higher mortality from all causes, as well as increased incidence of cancer, cardiovascular disease, and type 2 diabetes, even among people who exercise regularly, according to a meta-analysis published in the January 20 issue of the *Annals of Internal Medicine*. However, the analysis of 47 previously published articles also shows that the association between all-cause mortality and sedentary behavior is greatest among people who exercise the least.

TV

In 2013, 68% of 2034 Australian adults in an online survey thought it was appropriate to limit children's screen time to the recommended ≤2 h/day But most adults themselves spent >2 h watching TV and using the computer at home on work days (66%) and non-work days (88%).

Strategies people can use to reduce sitting time.
The target is to decrease sedentary time by two to three hours in a 12-hour day.
1. Monitor sitting times once we start counting, we're more likely to change our behavior
2. Set achievable goals and finding opportunities to incorporate greater physical activity -- and less time sitting -- into daily life:
   a. Work, stand up or move for one to three minutes every half hour; and when
   b. Leisure eg watching television, stand or exercise during commercials

Exercise and Brain Health
The aging process is associated with declines in brain function, including memory and how fast our brain processes information. Previous research has found that higher levels of cardiorespiratory fitness in older adults leads to better executive function in the brain, which helps with reasoning and problem solving. Higher cardiorespiratory fitness levels have also been found to increase brain volume in key brain regions and suggests that we can improve our brain health by changing our lifestyle even as we age.

Regular exercise critical for heart health, longevity
Small amounts of physical activity, including standing, are associated with a lower risk of cardiovascular disease, but more exercise leads to even greater reduction in risk of death from cardiovascular disease. Studies have shown that regular physical activity reduces a person's risk of death from cardiovascular disease; however, only half of U.S. adults meet the federally recommended guidelines of 150 minutes per week of moderate intensity exercise or 75 minutes per week of vigorous intensity exercise. Increasing the amount of moderate intensity exercise a person engages in results in increased reductions in cardiovascular disease mortality; however, the reductions in cardiovascular mortality benefits from vigorous intensity exercise do level out at a certain point.
There is no evidence for an upper limit to exercise-induced health benefits and all amounts of both moderate and vigorous intensity exercise result in a reduction of both all-cause and cardiovascular disease mortality compared to physical inactivity.
For cardiovascular disease patients, exercise can save lives, but one study showed that only 62 percent of heart attack patients were referred to cardiac rehabilitation at hospital discharge. Of those, just 23 percent attended more than one rehab session and only 5.4 percent completed more than 36 sessions.

Physical activity associated with lower risk for many cancers

In a study of 1.4 million participants higher levels of physical activity compared to lower levels were associated with lower risks of 13 of 26 cancers: esophageal adenocarcinoma (42 percent lower risk); liver (27 percent lower risk); lung (26 percent lower risk); kidney (23 percent lower risk); gastric cardia (22 percent lower risk); endometrial (21 percent lower risk); myeloid leukemia (20 percent lower risk); myeloma (17 percent lower risk); colon (16 percent lower risk); head and neck (15 percent lower risk), rectal (13 percent lower risk); bladder (13 percent lower risk); and breast (10 percent lower risk). Most of the associations remained regardless of body size or smoking history, according to the article. Overall, a higher level of physical activity was associated with a 7 percent lower risk of total cancer.

These findings underscore the importance of leisure-time physical activity as a potential risk reduction strategy to decrease the cancer burden in the United States and abroad. They demonstrate that high vs. low levels of physical activity engagement are associated with reduced risk of 13 cancer types (including 3 of the top 4 leading cancers among men and women worldwide). The widespread generalizability of these findings is reinforced by the suggestion that the associations persist regardless of BMI or smoking status.

The Exercise Hormone

Irisin, a hormone linked to the positive benefits of exercise, was discovered in 2012. This was exciting because scientists had potentially found one reason why exercise keeps us healthy. When irisin levels were increased in mice, their blood and metabolism improved. Results from human studies are still mixed as to what kinds of exercise raise irisin, but data suggest that high-intensity training protocols are particularly effective and further studies are necessary to fully understand how the hormone works in humans, specifically how it relates to brown and beige fat tissue and energy use.

CHAPTER 11.
INJURIES

* A top-class swimmer makes > 4000 overhead strokes in 1 training session, 800,000 in a season. Hence 60% have over-use injury of the shoulder.
* In 1 mile a 70 kg runner absorbs at least 200,000 kg of force - even the smallest problem often leads to overuse injuries of the legs and spine.
* ~ half of all injuries sustained in childhood & adolescence are the result of sporting activities & half of these due to overuse esp heavy training in the growing body
* Pain indicates injury. Do not continue through shin or shoulder pain, stop. Rest it. Then go back at a lighter level
* Women incur overuse injuries > men esp patellofemoral pain, stress fractures and lat epicondylitis due to anatomical differences
* Female Athlete Triad: disordered eating, amenorrhoea & osteoporosis

Overuse injuries of the M/S System.
* There has been a dramatic increase in overuse injuries in the last decade corresponding with endurance events being the rage
* When it feels like it's too much, it's too much," he said. "There is absolutely a point of diminishing returns.
* Disorientation, severe muscle cramps, cessation of sweating and dizziness are warning signs
* Extreme over-exercising can cause sleeplessness, blood poisoning, fractures or heart damage
* Pushing the body too far can cause intestinal bacteria to leak into the bloodstream, causing blood poisoning.
* A 2012 study also showed long-term endurance running may cause heart muscle scarring.
* Continual fatigue, decrease in performance, a sense of apathy or distraction are subtle signs of overtraining
* Jet Skis and Skidoos
* The continual pounding can see users compress their height by 2 cm.

Injuries In Older Exercisers
- Sport and recreational activities cause potentially preventable injuries
- Knowing what these injuries is the first step to preventing them:
- Men had more injuries than women
- Exercising caused 30% injuries to women
- Bicycling caused 17% injuries in men
- 27% of injuries were fractures. Women were more likely to suffer fractures than men
- When women had to do the same basic training as men in the British Army they had x 8 times the injuries
- A similar study in the US Army found women's injuries narrowed the gap as they got fitter

Common Injuries
Acute: Sprains, strains, tendinitis/osis (drugs), fractures (steroids), dislocations
Chronic: Rotator cuff, Ms overload, Stress #, Nerve Damage

Avoiding Injury - Weights
* Know what exercise & why
* Breathe - holding breath raises BP
* Balance & symmetry
* Appropriate weight - tired after 10 to 15 reps best
* Don't do too much - to fatigue and no more
* Don't rush - don't be too slow
* Rest - a days recovery for that muscle group
* Be consistent x3 / wk builds Muscles; x2 maintains
* Wear shoes
* Store weights properly - be careful picking up

Prevention
3 Types of Proven Interventions
1. Insoles – 50% reduction lower limb injuries
2. External joint supports – 50% reduction in ankle, wrist or knee injuries)

Multi-intervention training programs – 50% reduction in sports injuries

Danger: Don't Over-Exercise
Despite the recommendations of these studies it must be pointed out, yet again, that these are research statistics whereas, clinicians, myself included, see actual patients and see a different sample base – those who are ill and who, as such, are most likely not to have filled out these research statistics forms. To wit there is a definite danger in over-exercising in those prone to

heart disease. These need not be the fat and sedentary but often include the lean Tri-athlete who most assume must be healthy, but a Barcelona study found

- Cumulative heavy sports activity > 2000 hours or 35.5 hours a week or 5 hours a day had an odds ratio of 4.52 (more chance of getting Atrial Fibrillation, while being sedentary was 3.85
- Heavy exercisers had a sixfold increase for Atrial Fibrillaion compared with light to moderate exerciser

Resume
Walking, swimming and supervised yoga are the least injury exercises.

CHAPTER 12.
EXERCISE AND WEIGHT

Exercise is not very efficient for losing weight but is essential: Five times more energy is needed to get rid of fat than to get rid of muscle and so the body resists fat loss.

Exercise is important especially for maintaining weight loss long-term. One of its most useful contributions is that it minimizes the increases in hunger experienced from dieting. It does not cause an increase in hunger to the same extent as dieting, despite, if and when, it burns off the same reduction in calories.

In fact, hunger is reduced when exercising intensely, which may help to stave off hunger pangs while increasing the energy deficit.

Exercise has been touted by the soda-soft drink and fast-food industries as the healthy way to lose weight. The truth is the direct opposite. The people who drink sugary drinks and eat fast foods are invariably overweight.

30 minutes of jogging or swimming may burn off 350 cals but it is much easier to consume 350 less calories by not drinking soda / soft drinks or nonhungry junk food eating.

Most guidelines for obesity management recommend high exercise volumes, at 150 to 250 minutes/week and up to 60 minutes/day of moderate-intensity aerobic exercise. However, few people meet these guidelines.

Age Weight Gain
There is both an absolute gain in weight and also a relative percentage increase in fat between 40 and 50 years from 28% to 35% with central adiposity. Thereafter it is more stable.

The Good News
The good news is you can do this 30 minutes a day in six 5 minute bursts.

The Even Better News
The latest research suggests Interval training may result in greater weight loss than continuous exercise, with sprint interval training (SIT) the most effective: Just 40 seconds three times a week is enough and is the equivalent of running for 45 minutes.

Interval training was associated with a reduction in total absolute fat mass that was more than 28% greater than that seen with MOD, with the greatest reductions seen with SIT.

The advantage of interval training is that it can be performed by almost everyone, but participants have to know how to adapt it and calculate 'intensity' individually.

Live Longest recommends SIT and HIIPA plus Resistance Training
SIT: 40 seconds exercise bike three times a week
and
Resistance: Incidental Physical Activity – walking fast, taking the stairs until you puff.
Using the shopping for lifting weights.

To Lose Abdominal (Waist) Fat
Best exercise to lose abdominal fat (waist circumference) and build muscles is Weight Training (12 year study Harvard)

To reduce Visceral fat
Visceral fat is deep and accumulates around abdominal organs and is associated with metabolic problems / syndrome

Moderate exercise _brisk_ walking 30 min a day / 3 hr a week halts accumulation

45 min / day 5 days / week reduced it 3.4 to 6.9% pa while maintaining same calorie intake

High intensity (jogging 3 hrs / 20 miles a week) reduced it by 7% pa

Remaining sedentary gained 9% visceral fat in 6/12

Body burns calories to maintain basic subconscious essentials - breathing, circulation, organ function = BMR (Basal or Resting Metabolic Rate) – **see Book 4.**

* Aerobic exercise burns carbohydrates (Glycogen) or fat
* To burn fat choose a longer, moderate intensity exercise such as walking, swimming also see later studies
* Short term, high intensity (aerobic) such as 100m sprints, tend to burn glycogen

Again, SIT would seem to best preferable
Obviously, you should get medical clearance before proceeding. For a healthy young man, a sprint probably involves running at high velocities, but for a frail elder, slow walking might be enough. For individuals who

have knee problems and are not able to run, you can cycle or swim. If you have heart disease, you can walk at a controlled intensity. But, as above, a stationary bike would seem the overall best choice.

Regular physical activity is 'magic bullet' for pandemics of obesity, cardiovascular disease
Weight gain as well as being overweight or obese in middle age increase the risk for cardiovascular disease including heart attacks and stroke as well as type 2 diabetes, osteoarthritis and some common and fatal cancers such as colon cancer.

Starting in their 30s, Americans and many Europeans tend to gain between 1 and 3 pounds of body weight per year, and by 55, many are between 30 and 50 pounds overweight. This typical weight gain also is marked by an increase in adipose tissue mass and loss of lean body mass that accompanies an inactive lifestyle.

Modern inactive lifestyles seem to be important in the etiology of obesity
Physical activity confers important beneficial effects beyond body weight and include blood pressure, cholesterol, triglyceride, diabetes, heart attacks, strokes, colon cancer and possibly even breast and prostate cancers as well as arthritis, mood, energy, sleep and sex life. Lack of physical activity accounts for 22 percent of coronary heart disease, 22 percent of colon cancer, 18 percent of osteoporotic fractures, 12 percent of diabetes and hypertension, and five percent of breast cancer.

Brisk walking for only 20 minutes a day burns about 700 calories a week, results in a 30 to 40 percent reduced risk of coronary heart disease and can be performed even by the elderly. There is a need for increased awareness of the importance of resistance training as a valuable adjunct to regular aerobic activity such as brisk walking. Regular physical activity also should include resistance exercise such as lifting weights, which can even be safely performed in the elderly and in patients with heart failure. The maintenance or increase in lean body mass derived from lifting weights promotes an increase in the calories people burn at rest which adds a significant additional contribution to control of body weight. The general health benefits of resistance training for middle-aged and older adults are many, including the prevention or limitation of age-related sarcopenia, improved maintenance of muscle mass strength, and a decreased risk of osteoporosis-related bone fractures, falls, physical disability, and mortality

Finally, as to the importance of Resistance Training for Older Adults, a most complete "Position Statement From the National Strength and Conditioning Association" (USA), is available and highly recommended at 'The Journal of Strength & Conditioning Research': August 2019 - Volume 33 - Issue 8 - p 2019–2052 doi: 10.1519/JSC.0000000000000323

Best Exercise for Weight Loss
Comparing 18 different exercise regimes, regular jogging was the best type of exercise for managing obesity, according to five measures. Moreover, mountain climbing, walking, power walking, certain types of dancing, and long yoga practices also reduce BMI in individuals predisposed to obesity. Surprisingly, cycling, stretching exercises, swimming and Dance Dance Revolution did not counteract the genetic effects on obesity.

INDEX

A

Aging
  Changes 61–71
  Longevity 75–83, 187
    Life Expectancy 75–77
    The Blue Zones 80–81, 187
  Maintenance 85. See also Aging: Prevention
  Parental Responsibility 58
  Pathologic Aging 82
  Premature Aging 82. See also Illness & Injury: Premature Deaths & Disabilities
  Preparation 119–122
  Prevention 85, 86–87. See also Aging: Maintenance
  Successful Aging 57–60. See also Aging: Longevity
Alcohol 32, 33. See also Diet & Weight Loss
Alzheimer Disease. See Illness & Injury: Alzheimer Disease

B

C

Cancer. See Illness & Injury: Cancer
Cardiovascular Disease. See Illness & Injury: Cardiovascular
Cognitive Health. See Illness & Injury: Cognitive Health

D

Diabetes. See Illness & Injury: Endocrine

Diet & Weight Loss. See also Newtrition; See also Super-Mediterranean Diet; See also Exercise & Physical Activity; See also Food
  Behaviour 231
  Benefits 239
  Consequences 243
  Essentials 245
  Expectations 229
  Hints, Tricks & Good Advice 239
  Maintenance 237
  Mindfulness 234
  Mindlessness 234
  Motivation 233, 235
  Personalised 229
  Phytonutrients 23
  Recommendations 229
  Traps 238
Disability. See Illness & Injury
Drugs. See also Vitamins; See also Supplements
  Illicit Drugs 213
  Prescription Medicine 111–113, 117
  Tobacco 133. See also Illness & Injury: Respiratory

E

Endocrine Discrupting Chemicals (EDC). See Pollutants
Exercise & Physical Activity
  Aging 301
  Benefits 305–316
  Definitions 257–258
  Grades 257
  HIIPA 273–277, 279–295
  Injuries 317–319
  Measurement: METS 259
  METS. See Measurement: METS
  Motivation 269–271
  Over 65s 295–299
  Planning 267
  Programs 279–295. See also Exercise & Physical Activity: SIT; See also Exercise & Physical Activity: Resistance Training; See also Exercise & Physical Activity:

HIIPA; See also Exercise &
  Physical Activity: HIT
Resistance Training 279–295
SIT 279–295
Types 261–265
Weight Losss 321–324

F

Food. See also Diet & Weight Loss; See
    also Exercise & Physical Activity
  Best Breakfast Foods 19
  Worst Breakfast Foods 19
  Carbohydrates 49–51
  Eggs 48
  Macronutrient 23
  Meat 47–48
    Processed Meats 31, 32, 50
  Micronutrient 23
  Milk 46
  Processed Foods 32, 37–48. See
      also Food: Meat: Processed Meats
  Protein Shakes 34

G H

I

Illness & Injury

  Causes 64–65, 133
  Diagnosis 203–205, 207–211
  Treatment 203–205, 207–211
  Prevention 305–316
  Alzheimer Disease 34, 102–108, 214.
      See also Illness & Injury: Dementia
  Atherosclerosis 67. See also Illness &
      Injury: Cardiovascular
  Autism 28
  Cancer 27, 28, 31, 141, 143, 145, 146,
      213
  Cardiovascular 27, 28, 67, 141, 145,
      146, 204, 214. See also Illness &
      Injury: Atherosclerosis
  Cognitive Health. See also Illness &
      Injury: Alzheimer Disease; See
      also Illness & Injury: Dementia

  Aging 67, 95–99
    Memory 95–96
    Promoting 96
    Silver Tsunami Iom 96
  Dementia 67, 101–108, 214. See
      also Illness & Injury: Alzheimer
      Disease
  Endocrine 205
    Diabetes 27, 28, 141
  Falls 68
  Mental Health 90–94, 117–118, 141,
      143, 145, 146, 205, 213
  Musculoskeletal 147, 204
    Osteoarthritis 67, 141
    Osteoporosis 67, 141
    Spinal lordosis 67
  Nervous System 204
  Obesity 133, 225–228
  Physical Health
    Aging 63–64, 66–67, 88–90, 123–126,
        189
  Premature Deaths & Disabilities 133–
      173, 181–182, 193–194, 195–196.
      See also Illness & Injury: Physical
      Health; See also Men's Health; See
      also Women's Health
    Health Criteria 183–184
  Prevalent Health Problems 197–199
  Respiratory 143, 145, 146, 204
    Asthma 141
  Sarcopenia 68, 257, 301
  Sex 117
  Skin 67
  Stroke 141
  Taste 67

J

K

Keto Diet
  230

L

M

Memory. See Illness & Injury: Cognitive Health
Men's Health 157, 159–160, 161–164, 165–170, 171–173, 195–196, 205, 211. See also Illness & Injury: Premature Deaths & Disabilities
Mental Health. See Illness & Injury: Mental Health
Microwave 109. See also Diet & Weight Loss; See also Pollutants

N

Newtrition 18, 20, 41. See also Super-Mediterranean Diet

O

Obesity. See Illness & Injury: Obesity

P

Paleo Diet 230
Physical Activity. See Exercise & Physical Activity
Physical Health. See Illness & Injury: Physical Health
Phytonutrients. See Diet & Weight Loss
Plant-based Diet. See Diet & Weight Loss: Phytonutrients
Pollutants 109
Premature Death. See Illness & Injury: Premature Deaths & Disabilities
Premature Disabilities. See Illness & Injury: Premature Deaths & Disabilities

Q R

S

Sex 115–118
Sleep
  Aging 88
Smoking. See Drugs: Tobacco
Stress 99
Super-Mediterranean Diet 15, 17. See also Newtrition

Supplements iii, vii, 34, 113. See also Vitamins

T U

V

Vitamins iii, vii, 28, 113. See also Supplements

W

Weight Loss. See Diet & Weight Loss
Women's Health 139, 141, 143, 145–148, 149–152, 153–156, 195–196, 205, 211. See also Illness & Injury: Premature Deaths & Disabilities

X Y Z

**SCAN TO VIEW THE
FULL UNCONDENSED EDITIONS:**

1. NEWTRITION
2. SUCCESSFUL AGING
3. WHAT'S GOING TO KILL YOU (THIS YEAR)
4. SLIM 4 LIFE

livelongest.com.au

Pacific Medical Laboratories PO Box 6144

www.ingramcontent.com/pod-product-compliance
Lightning Source LLC
Chambersburg PA
CBHW070906030426
42336CB00014BA/2312